UCV

BLACKWELL

UNDERGROUND CLINICAL VIGNETTES

PHARMACOLOGY, 4E

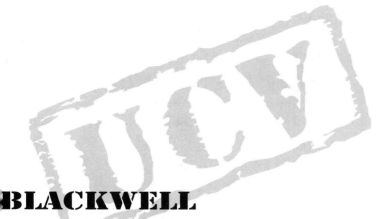

BLACKWELL

UNDERGROUND CLINICAL VIGNETTES

PHARMACOLOGY, 4E

VIKAS BHUSHAN, MD
Series Editor
University of California, San Francisco, Class of 1991
Diagnostic Radiologist

VISHAL PALL, MD MPH
Series Editor
Internist and Preventive Medicine Specialist
Government Medical College, Chandigarh – Panjab University – India, Class of 1997
Graduate School of Biomedical Sciences at UTMB Galveston, MPH, Class of 2004

TAO LE, MD
University of California, San Francisco, Class of 1996

ALIREZA KHAZAEIZADEH, MD
Shiraz University School of Medicine, Class of 1995
Associate Professor, Department of Biochemistry, St. Luke's
University School of Medicine

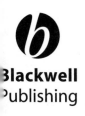

Blackwell
Publishing

© 2005 by Blackwell Publishing

Blackwell Publishing, Inc., 350 Main Street, Malden, Massachusetts 02148-5018, USA
Blackwell Publishing Ltd, 9600 Garsington Road, Oxford OX4 2DQ, UK
Blackwell Publishing Asia Pty Ltd, 550 Swanston Street, Carlton, Victoria 3053, Australia

05 06 07 08 5 4 3 2 1

ISBN-13: 978-1-4051-0417-3
ISBN-10: 1-4051-0417-1

Library of Congress Cataloging-in-Publication Data

Pharmacology / Vikas Bhushan . . . [et al.]. — 4th ed.
    p. ; cm. — (Blackwell underground clinical vignettes)
  ISBN-13: 978-1-4051-0417-3 (pbk. : alk. paper)
  ISBN-10: 1-4051-0417-1 (pbk. : alk. paper)   1. Clinical pharmacology—Case studies.
2. Physicians—Licenses—United States—Examinations—Study guides.
  [DNLM: 1. Pharmacology—Case Reports.   2. Pharmacology—Problems and Exercises. QV 18.2
P5353 2005] I. Bhushan, Vikas. II. Series: Blackwell's underground clinical vignettes.

  RM301.28.P48 2005
  615′.1′076—dc22

                                                                                    2005003550

A catalogue record for this title is available from the British Library

Acquisitions: Nancy Anastasi Duffy
Development/Production: Jennifer Kowalewski
Cover and Interior design: Leslie Haimes
Typesetter: Graphicraft in Quarry Bay, Hong Kong
Printed and bound by Capital City Press in Berlin, VT

For further information on Blackwell Publishing, visit our website:
www.blackwellmedstudent.com

NOTICE
The indications and dosages of all drugs in this book have been recommended in the medical literature
and conform to the practices of the general community. The medications described do not necessarily
have specific approval by the Food and Drug Administration for use in the diseases and dosages for
which they are recommended. The package insert for each drug should be consulted for use and dosage
as approved by the FDA. Because standards for usage change, it is advisable to keep abreast of revised
recommendations, particularly those concerning new drugs.

The authors of this volume have taken care that the information contained herein is accurate and compatible with the standards generally accepted at the time of publication. Nevertheless, it is difficult to
ensure that all the information given is entirely accurate for all circumstances. The publisher and
authors do not guarantee the contents of this book and disclaim any liability, loss, or damage incurred
as a consequence, directly or indirectly, of the use and application of any of the contents of this volume.

The publisher's policy is to use permanent paper from mills that operate a sustainable forestry policy
and which has been manufactured from pulp processed using acid-free and elementary chlorine-free
practices. Furthermore, the publisher ensures that the text paper and cover board used have met
acceptable environmental accreditation standards.

CONTENTS

HEMATOLOGY/ONCOLOGY

IMMUNOLOGY

INFECTIOUS DISEASE

NEPHROLOGY/UROLOGY

NEUROLOGY

ORTHOPEDICS

PSYCHOPHARMACOLOGY

CONTRIBUTORS

Hoang Nguyen, MD, MBA
Northwestern University, Class of 2001

Joseph Hastings
David Geffen School of Medicine at UCLA, Class of 2006
UCLA School of Public Health, MPH, Class of 2006

M. Houman Fekrazad, MD
Shiraz University School of Medicine, Class of 1994
Resident in Internal Medicine, Carraway Methodist Medical Center, Birmingham AL

Sameer Sheth, PhD
David Geffen School of Medicine at UCLA, Class of 2005
Faculty Reviewer

Bertram Katzung, MD, PhD
Professor Emeritus of Pharmacology, UCSF School of Medicine

ACKNOWLEDGMENTS

Throughout the production of this book, we have had the support of many friends and colleagues. Special thanks to our support team including Andrea Fellows, Anastasia Anderson, Srishti Gupta, Anu Gupta, Mona Pall, Jonathan Kirsch and Chirag Amin. For prior contributions we thank Gianni Le Nguyen, Tarun Mathur, Alex Grimm, Sonia Santos and Elizabeth Sanders.

For submitting comments, corrections, editing, proofreading, and assistance across all of the vignette titles in all editions, we collectively thank:

Tara Adamovich, Carolyn Alexander, Kris Alden, Henry E. Aryan, Lynman Bacolor, Natalie Barteneva, Dean Bartholomew, Debashish Behera, Sumit Bhatia, Sanjay Bindra, Dave Brinton, Julianne Brown, Alexander Brownie, Tamara Callahan, David Canes, Bryan Casey, Aaron Caughey, Hebert Chen, Jonathan Cheng, Arnold Cheung, Arnold Chin, Simion Chiosea, Yoon Cho, Samuel Chung, Gretchen Conant, Vladimir Coric, Christopher Cosgrove, Ronald Cowan, Karekin R. Cunningham, A. Sean Dalley, Rama Dandamudi, Sunit Das, Ryan Armando Dave, John David, Emmanuel de la Cruz, Robert DeMello, Navneet Dhillon, Sharmila Dissanaike, David Donson, Adolf Etchegaray, Alea Eusebio, Jose M. Fierro, Priscilla A. Frase, David Frenz, Kristin Gaumer, Yohannes Gebreegziabher, Anil Gehi, Abby Geltemeyer, Tony George, L.M. Gotanco, Parul Goyal, Alex Grimm, Rajeev Gupta, Ahmad Halim, Sue Hall, David Hasselbacher, Tamra Heimert, Michelle Higley, Dan Hoit, Eric Jackson, Tim Jackson, Sundar Jayaraman, Pei-Ni Jone, Aarchan Joshi, Rajni K Jutla, Faiyaz Kapadi, Seth Karp, Aaron S. Kesselheim, Sana Khan, Andrew Pin-wei Ko, Francis Kong, Paul Konitzky, Warren S. Krackov, Benjamin H.S. Lau, Ann LaCasce, Connie Lee, Scott Lee, Guillermo Lehmann, Kevin Leung, Paul Levett, Warren Levinson, Eric Ley, Ken Lin, Pavel Lobanov, J. Mark Maddox, Aram Mardian, Samir Mehta, Gil Melmed, Joe Messina, Robert Mosca, Michael Murphy, Vivek Nandkarni, Siva Narayanan, Carvell Nguyen, Linh Nguyen, Deanna Nobleza, Craig Nodurft, George Noumi, Darin T. Okuda, Adam L. Palance, Paul Pamphrus, Jinha Park, Sonny Patel, Ricardo Pietrobon, Riva L. Rahl, Aashita Randeria, Rachan Reddy, Beatriu Reig, Marilou Reyes, Jeremy Richmon, Ta Roe, Rick Roller, Rajiv Roy, Diego Ruiz, Anthony Russell, Sanjay Sahgal, Urmimala Sarkar, John Schilling, Isabell Schmitt, Daren Schuhmacher, Sonal Shah, Mae Sheikh-All, Edie Shen, Justin Smith, Vipal Soni, John Stulak, Lillian Su, Julie Sundaram, Rita Suri, Seth Sweetser, Antonio Talayero, Merita Tan, Mark Tanaka, Eric Taylor, Jess Thompson, Ind Trehan, Raymond Turner, Okafo Uchenna, Eric Uyguanco, Richa Varma, John Wages, Alan Wang, Eunice Wang, Andy Weiss, Amy Williams, Brian Yang, Hany Zaky, Ashraf Zamar and David Zipf.

Please let us know if your name has been missed or misspelled and we will be happy to make the update in the next edition.

For generously contributing images to the entire Underground Clinical Vignette Step 1 series, we collectively thank the staff at Blackwell Publishing in Oxford, Boston, and Berlin as well as:

- Axford, J. Medicine. Osney Mead: Blackwell Science Ltd, 1996. Figures 2.14, 2.15, 2.16, 2.27, 2.28, 2.31, 2.35, 2.36, 2.38, 2.43, 2.65a, 2.65b, 2.65c, 2.103b, 2.105b, 3.20b, 3.21, 8.27, 8.27b, 8.77b, 8.77c, 10.81b, 10.96a, 12.28a, 14.6, 14.16, 14.50.

Bannister B, Begg N, Gillespie S. Infectious Disease, 2nd Edition. Osney Mead: Blackwell Science Ltd, 2000. Figures 2.8, 3.4, 5.28, 18.10, W5.32, W5.6.

Berg D. Advanced Clinical Skills and Physical Diagnosis. Blackwell Science Ltd., 1999. Figures 7.10, 7.12, 7.13, 7.2, 7.3, 7.7, 7.8, 7.9, 8.1, 8.2, 8.4, 8.5, 9.2, 10.2, 11.3, 11.5, 12.6.

Cuschieri A, Hennessy TPJ, Greenhalgh RM, Rowley DA, Grace PA. Clinical Surgery. Osney Mead: Blackwell Science Ltd, 1996. Figures 13.19, 18.22, 18.33.

Gillespie SH, Bamford K. *Medical Microbiology and Infection at a Glance.* Osney Mead.: Blackwell Science Ltd, 2000, Figures 20, 23.

Ginsberg L. Lecture Notes on Neurology, 7th Edition. Osney Mead: Blackwell Science Ltd, 1999. Figures 12.3, 18.3, 18.3b.

Elliott T, Hastings M, Desselberger U. Lecture Notes on Medical Microbiology, 3rd Edition. Osney Mead: Blackwell Science Ltd, 1997. Figures 2, 5, 7, 8, 9, 11, 12, 14, 15, 16, 17, 19, 20, 25, 26, 27, 29, 30, 34, 35, 52.

Mehta AB, Hoffbrand AV. Haematology at a Glance. Osney Mead: Blackwell Science Ltd, 2000. Figures 22.1, 22.2, 22.3.

HOW TO USE THIS BOOK

This series was originally developed to address the increasing number of clinical vignette questions on medical examinations, including the USMLE Step 1 and Step 2.

Each UCV 1 book uses a series of approximately 100 "supra-prototypical" cases as a way to condense testable facts and associations. The clinical vignettes in this series are designed to give added emphasis to pathogenesis, epidemiology, management and complications. Although each case tends to present all the signs, symptoms, and diagnostic findings for a particular illness, **patients generally will not present with such a "complete" picture either clinically or on a medical examination.** Cases are not meant to simulate a potential real patient or an exam vignette. **All the boldfaced "buzzwords" are for learning purposes** and are not necessarily expected to be found in any one patient with the disease.

Definitions of selected important terms are placed within the vignettes in (small caps) in parentheses. Other parenthetical remarks often refer to the pathophysiology or mechanism of disease. The format should also help students learn to present cases succinctly during oral "bullet" presentations on clinical rotations. The cases are meant to serve as a condensed review, not as a primary reference. The information provided in this book has been prepared with a great deal of thought and careful research. This book should not, however, be considered as your sole source of information. Corrections, suggestions and submissions of new cases are encouraged and will be acknowledged and incorporated when appropriate in future editions.

We hope that you find the *Blackwell Underground Clinical Vignettes* series informative and useful. We welcome feedback and suggestions you have about this book, or any published by Blackwell Publishing.

Please e-mail us at medfeedback@bos.blackwellpublishing.com.

ABBREVIATIONS

ABGs	arterial blood gases
ABPA	allergic bronchopulmonary aspergillosis
ACA	anticardiolipin antibody
ACE	angiotensin-converting enzyme
ACL	anterior cruciate ligament
ACTH	adrenocorticotropic hormone
AD	adjustment disorder
ADA	adenosine deaminase
ADD	attention deficit disorder
ADH	antidiuretic hormone
ADHD	attention deficit hyperactivity disorder
ADP	adenosine diphosphate
AFO	ankle-foot orthosis
AFP	α-fetoprotein
AIDS	acquired immunodeficiency syndrome
ALL	acute lymphocytic leukemia
ALS	amyotrophic lateral sclerosis
ALT	alanine aminotransferase
AML	acute myelogenous leukemia
ANA	antinuclear antibody
Angio	angiography
AP	anteroposterior
APKD	adult polycystic kidney disease
aPTT	activated partial thromboplastin time
ARDS	adult respiratory distress syndrome
5-ASA	5-aminosalicylic acid
ASCA	antibodies to *Saccharomyces cerevisiae*
ASO	antistreptolysin O
AST	aspartate aminotransferase
ATLL	adult T-cell leukemia/lymphoma
ATPase	adenosine triphosphatase
AV	arteriovenous, atrioventricular
AZT	azidothymidine (zidovudine)
BAL	British antilewisite (dimercaprol)
BCG	bacille Calmette-Guérin
BE	barium enema
BP	blood pressure
BPH	benign prostatic hypertrophy
BUN	blood urea nitrogen
CABG	coronary artery bypass grafting
CAD	coronary artery disease
CaEDTA	calcium edetate
CALLA	common acute lymphoblastic leukemia antigen
cAMP	cyclic adenosine monophosphate
C-ANCA	cytoplasmic antineutrophil cytoplasmic antibody
CBC	complete blood count

CBD	common bile duct
CCU	cardiac care unit
CD	cluster of differentiation
2-CdA	2-chlorodeoxyadenosine
CEA	carcinoembryonic antigen
CFTR	cystic fibrosis transmembrane conductance regulator
cGMP	cyclic guanosine monophosphate
CHF	congestive heart failure
CK	creatine kinase
CK-MB	creatine kinase, MB fraction
CLL	chronic lymphocytic leukemia
CML	chronic myelogenous leukemia
CMV	cytomegalovirus
CN	cranial nerve
CNS	central nervous system
COPD	chronic obstructive pulmonary disease
COX	cyclooxygenase
CP	cerebellopontine
CPAP	continuous positive airway pressure
CPK	creatine phosphokinase
CPPD	calcium pyrophosphate dihydrate
CPR	cardiopulmonary resuscitation
CREST	calcinosis, Raynaud's phenomenon, esophageal involvement, sclerodactyly, telangiectasia (syndrome)
CRP	C-reactive protein
CSF	cerebrospinal fluid
CSOM	chronic suppurative otitis media
CT	cardiac transplant, computed tomography
CVA	cerebrovascular accident
CXR	chest x-ray
d4T	didehydrodeoxythymidine (stavudine)
DCS	decompression sickness
DDH	developmental dysplasia of the hip
ddI	dideoxyinosine (didanosine)
DES	diethylstilbestrol
DEXA	dual-energy x-ray absorptiometry
DHEAS	dehydroepiandrosterone sulfate
DIC	disseminated intravascular coagulation
DIF	direct immunofluorescence
DIP	distal interphalangeal (joint)
DKA	diabetic ketoacidosis
DL_{CO}	diffusing capacity of carbon monoxide
DMSA	2,3-dimercaptosuccinic acid
DNA	deoxyribonucleic acid
DNase	deoxyribonuclease
2,3-DPG	2,3-diphosphoglycerate

dsDNA	double-stranded DNA
DSM	Diagnostic and Statistical Manual
dsRNA	double-stranded RNA
DTP	diphtheria, tetanus, pertussis (vaccine)
DTPA	diethylenetriamine-penta-acetic acid
DTs	delirium tremens
DVT	deep venous thrombosis
EBV	Epstein-Barr virus
ECG	electrocardiography
Echo	echocardiography
ECM	erythema chronicum migrans
ECT	electroconvulsive therapy
EEG	electroencephalography
EF	ejection fraction, elongation factor
EGD	esophagogastroduodenoscopy
EHEC	enterohemorrhagic *E. coli*
EIA	enzyme immunoassay
ELISA	enzyme-linked immunosorbent assay
EM	electron microscopy
EMG	electromyography
ENT	ears, nose, and throat
EPVE	early prosthetic valve endocarditis
ER	emergency room
ERCP	endoscopic retrograde cholangiopancreatography
ERT	estrogen replacement therapy
ESR	erythrocyte sedimentation rate
ETEC	enterotoxigenic *E. coli*
EtOH	ethanol
FAP	familial adenomatous polyposis
FEV_1	forced expiratory volume in 1 second
FH	familial hypercholesterolemia
FNA	fine-needle aspiration
FSH	follicle-stimulating hormone
FTA-ABS	fluorescent treponemal antibody absorption test
FVC	forced vital capacity
G6PD	glucose-6-phosphate dehydrogenase
GABA	gamma-aminobutyric acid
GERD	gastroesophageal reflux disease
GFR	glomerular filtration rate
GGT	gamma-glutamyltransferase
GH	growth hormone
GI	gastrointestinal
GnRH	gonadotropin-releasing hormone
GU	genitourinary
GVHD	graft-versus-host disease
HAART	highly active antiretroviral therapy

HAV	hepatitis A virus
Hb	hemoglobin
HbA-1C	hemoglobin A-1C
HBsAg	hepatitis B surface antigen
HBV	hepatitis B virus
hCG	human chorionic gonadotropin
HCO_3	bicarbonate
Hct	hematocrit
HCV	hepatitis C virus
HDL	high-density lipoprotein
HDL-C	high-density lipoprotein-cholesterol
HEENT	head, eyes, ears, nose, and throat (exam)
HELLP	hemolysis, elevated LFTs, low platelets (syndrome)
HFMD	hand, foot, and mouth disease
HGPRT	hypoxanthine-guanine phosphoribosyltransferase
5-HIAA	5-hydroxyindoleacetic acid
HIDA	hepato-iminodiacetic acid (scan)
HIV	human immunodeficiency virus
HLA	human leukocyte antigen
HMG-CoA	hydroxymethylglutaryl-coenzyme A
HMP	hexose monophosphate
HPI	history of present illness
HPV	human papillomavirus
HR	heart rate
HRIG	human rabies immune globulin
HRS	hepatorenal syndrome
HRT	hormone replacement therapy
HSG	hysterosalpingography
HSV	herpes simplex virus
HTLV	human T-cell leukemia virus
HUS	hemolytic-uremic syndrome
HVA	homovanillic acid
ICP	intracranial pressure
ICU	intensive care unit
ID/CC	identification and chief complaint
IDDM	insulin-dependent diabetes mellitus
IFA	immunofluorescent antibody
Ig	immunoglobulin
IGF	insulin-like growth factor
IHSS	idiopathic hypertrophic subaortic stenosis
IM	intramuscular
IMA	inferior mesenteric artery
INH	isoniazid
INR	International Normalized Ratio
IP_3	inositol 1,4,5-triphosphate
IPF	idiopathic pulmonary fibrosis

ITP	idiopathic thrombocytopenic purpura
IUD	intrauterine device
IV	intravenous
IVC	inferior vena cava
IVIG	intravenous immunoglobulin
IVP	intravenous pyelography
JRA	juvenile rheumatoid arthritis
JVP	jugular venous pressure
KOH	potassium hydroxide
KUB	kidney, ureter, bladder
LCM	lymphocytic choriomeningitis
LDH	lactate dehydrogenase
LDL	low-density lipoprotein
LE	lupus erythematosus (cell)
LES	lower esophageal sphincter
LFTs	liver function tests
LH	luteinizing hormone
LMN	lower motor neuron
LP	lumbar puncture
LPVE	late prosthetic valve endocarditis
L/S	lecithin-sphingomyelin (ratio)
LSD	lysergic acid diethylamide
LT	labile toxin
LV	left ventricular
LVH	left ventricular hypertrophy
Lytes	electrolytes
Mammo	mammography
MAO	monoamine oxidase (inhibitor)
MCP	metacarpophalangeal (joint)
MCTD	mixed connective tissue disorder
MCV	mean corpuscular volume
MEN	multiple endocrine neoplasia
MI	myocardial infarction
MIBG	meta-iodobenzylguanidine (radioisotope)
MMR	measles, mumps, rubella (vaccine)
MPGN	membranoproliferative glomerulonephritis
MPS	mucopolysaccharide
MPTP	1-methyl-4-phenyl-tetrahydropyridine
MR	magnetic resonance (imaging)
mRNA	messenger ribonucleic acid
MRSA	methicillin-resistant S. aureus
MTP	metatarsophalangeal (joint)
NAD	nicotinamide adenine dinucleotide
NADP	nicotinamide adenine dinucleotide phosphate
NADPH	reduced nicotinamide adenine dinucleotide phosphate
NF	neurofibromatosis

NIDDM	non-insulin-dependent diabetes mellitus
NNRTI	non-nucleoside reverse transcriptase inhibitor
NO	nitric oxide
NPO	nil per os (nothing by mouth)
NSAID	nonsteroidal anti-inflammatory drug
Nuc	nuclear medicine
NYHA	New York Heart Association
OB	obstetric
OCD	obsessive-compulsive disorder
OCPs	oral contraceptive pills
OR	operating room
PA	posteroanterior
PABA	para-aminobenzoic acid
PAN	polyarteritis nodosa
P-ANCA	perinuclear antineutrophil cytoplasmic antibody
Pa_{O_2}	partial pressure of oxygen in arterial blood
PAS	periodic acid Schiff
PAT	paroxysmal atrial tachycardia
PBS	peripheral blood smear
P_{CO_2}	partial pressure of carbon dioxide
PCOM	posterior communicating (artery)
PCOS	polycystic ovarian syndrome
PCP	phencyclidine
PCR	polymerase chain reaction
PCT	porphyria cutanea tarda
PCTA	percutaneous coronary transluminal angioplasty
PCV	polycythemia vera
PDA	patent ductus arteriosus
PDGF	platelet-derived growth factor
PE	physical exam
PEFR	peak expiratory flow rate
PEG	polyethylene glycol
PEPCK	phosphoenolpyruvate carboxykinase
PET	positron emission tomography
PFTs	pulmonary function tests
PID	pelvic inflammatory disease
PIP	proximal interphalangeal (joint)
PKU	phenylketonuria
PMDD	premenstrual dysphoric disorder
PML	progressive multifocal leukoencephalopathy
PMN	polymorphonuclear (leukocyte)
PNET	primitive neuroectodermal tumor
PNH	paroxysmal nocturnal hemoglobinuria
P_{O_2}	partial pressure of oxygen
PPD	purified protein derivative (of tuberculosis)
PPH	primary postpartum hemorrhage

PRA	panel reactive antibody
PROM	premature rupture of membranes
PSA	prostate-specific antigen
PSS	progressive systemic sclerosis
PT	prothrombin time
PTH	parathyroid hormone
PTSD	post-traumatic stress disorder
PTT	partial thromboplastin time
PUVA	psoralen ultraviolet A
PVC	premature ventricular contraction
RA	rheumatoid arthritis
RAIU	radioactive iodine uptake
RAST	radioallergosorbent test
RBC	red blood cell
REM	rapid eye movement
RES	reticuloendothelial system
RFFIT	rapid fluorescent focus inhibition test
RFTs	renal function tests
RHD	rheumatic heart disease
RNA	ribonucleic acid
RNP	ribonucleoprotein
RPR	rapid plasma reagin
RR	respiratory rate
RSV	respiratory syncytial virus
RUQ	right upper quadrant
RV	residual volume
Sao_2	oxygen saturation in arterial blood
SBFT	small bowel follow-through
SCC	squamous cell carcinoma
SCID	severe combined immunodeficiency
SERM	selective estrogen receptor modulator
SGOT	serum glutamic-oxaloacetic transaminase
SIADH	syndrome of inappropriate antidiuretic hormone
SIDS	sudden infant death syndrome
SLE	systemic lupus erythematosus
SMA	superior mesenteric artery
SSPE	subacute sclerosing panencephalitis
SSRI	selective serotonin reuptake inhibitor
ST	stable toxin
STD	sexually transmitted disease
T2W	T2-weighted (MRI)
T_3	triiodothyronine
T_4	thyroxine
TAH-BSO	total abdominal hysterectomy–bilateral salpingo-oophorectomy
TB	tuberculosis
TCA	tricyclic antidepressant

TCC	transitional cell carcinoma
TDT	terminal deoxytransferase
TFTs	thyroid function tests
TGF	transforming growth factor
THC	tetrahydrocannabinol
TIA	transient ischemic attack
TLC	total lung capacity
TMP-SMX	trimethoprim-sulfamethoxazole
tPA	tissue plasminogen activator
TP-HA	*Treponema pallidum* hemagglutination assay
TPP	thiamine pyrophosphate
TRAP	tartrate-resistant acid phosphatase
tRNA	transfer ribonucleic acid
TSH	thyroid-stimulating hormone
TSS	toxic shock syndrome
TTP	thrombotic thrombocytopenic purpura
TURP	transurethral resection of the prostate
TXA	thromboxane A
UA	urinalysis
UDCA	ursodeoxycholic acid
UGI	upper GI
UPPP	uvulopalatopharyngoplasty
URI	upper respiratory infection
US	ultrasound
UTI	urinary tract infection
UV	ultraviolet
VDRL	Venereal Disease Research Laboratory
VIN	vulvar intraepithelial neoplasia
VIP	vasoactive intestinal polypeptide
VLDL	very low density lipoprotein
VMA	vanillylmandelic acid
V/Q	ventilation/perfusion (ratio)
VRE	vancomycin-resistant enterococcus
VS	vital signs
VSD	ventricular septal defect
vWF	von Willebrand's factor
VZV	varicella-zoster virus
WAGR	Wilms' tumor, aniridia, genitourinary abnormalities, mental retardation (syndrome)
WBC	white blood cell
WHI	Women's Health Initiative
WPW	Wolff-Parkinson-White syndrome
XR	x-ray
ZN	Ziehl-Neelsen (stain)

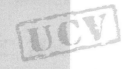

CARDIOLOGY

CASE 1

ID/CC

A 45-year-old female complains of **fatigue**, headache, dizziness, dry cough, **shortness of breath**, and **unexplained anxiety**.

HPI

She has been receiving warfarin and **amiodarone** for 1 year for treatment of chronic paroxysmal atrial fibrillation.

PE

VS: **bradycardia (HR 55)**; BP normal; no fever. PE: well hydrated, conscious, and oriented; no neck masses or bruit; **diffuse crackling sounds and wheezes** in both lung fields, predominantly in bases; abdominal and neurologic exams normal; violaceous skin discoloration in sun-exposed areas.

Labs

ECG: **prolonged Q-T interval** and QRS duration. **AST and ALT moderately elevated**; decreased TSH; increased free T_3 and T_4.

Imaging

CXR: bilateral interstitial infiltrates (incipient pulmonary fibrosis).

Treatment

Discontinue amiodarone; monitor Q-T interval until normal; steroids may be indicated for pulmonary toxicity; monitor LFTs and TFTs until they normalize after cessation of amiodarone use.

Discussion

Amiodarone is a class III antiarrhythmic drug. Adverse reactions require careful monitoring and include **thyroid dysfunction** (both hypo- and hyperthyroidism), **constipation, hepatocellular necrosis,** and **pulmonary fibrosis**, which may be fatal. It may also produce **bradycardia and heart block** in susceptible individuals. Amiodarone has a **long half-life**, so if toxicity occurs, it persists long after the drug has been discontinued. Amiodarone **increases the blood levels** of digoxin, phenytoin, and warfarin.

amiodarone side effects

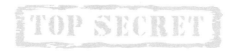

TOP SECRET

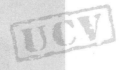

CASE 2

ID/CC

A 54-year-old obese male who is the owner of a chain of fast-food restaurants is brought to the ER after **fainting at work**; earlier in the morning he complained of **dizziness and dyspnea**.

HPI

He had been having episodes of acute, severe retrosternal chest pain associated with exercise or stress (ANGINA PECTORIS) for over 2 years and is taking **propranolol**.

PE

VS: **hypotension (BP 85/60); bradycardia** (HR 52); no fever. PE: patient is conscious; lung fields have **scattered wheezes** (BRONCHOSPASM); no hepatosplenomegaly or peritoneal signs.

Labs

ECG: QRS normal, but **P-R interval increased** (FIRST-DEGREE AV BLOCK).

Treatment

Treat bradycardia with atropine or epinephrine. Treat **bronchospasm** with bronchodilators. Treat hypotension with fluids and norepinephrine. Glucagon can be life-saving.

Discussion

Propranolol is a competitive nonselective beta-blocker that acts at both β_1 and β_2 receptors. β_2 receptors are found in bronchiolar and vascular smooth muscle. Uses include management of hypertension and tachyarrhythmias, hypertrophic cardiomyopathy, prevention of angina and migraines, reduction of mortality after myocardial infarction, and treatment of glaucoma and hyperthyroidism. Overdose can present with cardiac conduction disturbances, severe CNS toxicity (seizures, coma), and hyperkalemia.

beta-blocker overdose

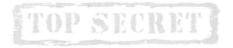

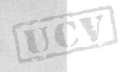

ID/CC

A 62-year-old female is referred to a pulmonary medicine specialist by her family physician because of a **chronic dry cough** that has been **unresponsive to medications**.

HPI

On careful, directed questioning, the specialist discovers that she had been taking **captopril** for hypertension for 3 years. She also complains of **taste changes** and a **rash** on her chest and lower legs.

PE

VS: normal. PE: no lymphadenopathy; funduscopic exam reveals grade I hypertensive retinopathy; discrete nonpruritic maculopapular **rash** on legs and chest.

Labs

Serum **renin increased; angiotensin II decreased**. Lytes: hyperkalemia. CBC/PFTs: normal. LFTs: normal. UA: mild **proteinuria**.

Imaging

CXR: no signs of COPD, neoplasm, or other pathology that would account for cough.

Treatment

Aspirin, nifedipine, or cromolyn may decrease cough. However, it may be necessary to switch to another antihypertensive. **Losartan** is an alternative agent that blocks the binding of angiotensin II to its receptor and does not cause cough.

Discussion

Captopril is an ACE inhibitor and thus reduces levels of angiotensin II and prevents the inactivation of bradykinin (a potent vasodilator). It is used to treat hypertension, CHF, and diabetic renal disease. It is **contraindicated in pregnancy** because of fetotoxicity; other side effects are **cough, hypotension, taste changes, rash, proteinuria, hyperkalemia, angioedema**, and **neutropenia**.

captopril side effects

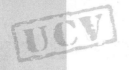

CASE 4

ID/CC
A 54-year-old white female complains of intermittent **nausea and vomiting, headaches, lethargy,** and **confusion** over the past 3 months.

HPI
She describes objects as **appearing yellow** to her. She has a history of heart failure with **chronic digoxin** use as well as **diuretics** (may induce hypokalemia).

PE
VS: **bradycardia** (HR 48); BP normal; no fever. PE: in no acute distress; slight increase in JVP; S3 present; rales at lung bases; mild hepatomegaly; ankle edema.

Labs
CBC: normal. Lytes: **hypokalemia.** Elevated BUN; elevated creatinine. ECG: **second-degree AV block with AV junctional rhythm.** Elevated serum digoxin level.

Imaging
CXR: moderate enlargement of the heart (due to long-standing CHF); no signs of lung infection.

Treatment
Lower and space apart the dose. Correct hypokalemia. Digoxin-specific Fab antibody fragments.

Discussion
Digoxin is a cardiac glycoside that inhibits the Na-K ATP-ase of cell membranes, causing an increase in intracellular sodium that results in an elevation in the intracellular calcium level, thereby causing positive inotropy. **Renal failure may precipitate toxicity at normal therapeutic doses** (excretion is decreased). Hypokalemia is a frequent predisposing factor for toxicity. ECG changes may vary widely; AV conduction disturbances, such as PAT with block, are characteristic, as are bigeminy, bradycardia, and flattened T waves.

digitalis intoxication

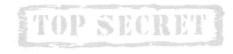

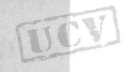

ID/CC   An anesthesiologist is summoned into the OR when a 34-year-old male undergoing a **routine hernia repair** begins to have **seizures**.

HPI   The surgeon was chatting with the chief resident while injecting **lidocaine** subcutaneously for a local anesthetic repair when the patient suddenly started having slurred speech, tremors, and **tonic-clonic convulsions** (lidocaine was inadvertently injected systemically into the inferior epigastric vessels).

PE   Lips and fingertips blue (CYANOSIS); patient **biting his tongue**; eyes rolled inward; spastic extremities and spine with shaking movements during intervals.

Labs   There was no time to take blood samples.

Treatment Control seizures with IV diazepam or barbiturates. Intubate, oxygenate, and ventilate in anticipation of second phase (respiratory depression).

Discussion Lidocaine is an amide that blocks sodium channels, primarily in rapidly firing cells such as those in the myocardium, in pain fibers, and in the CNS. Overdosage occurs with inadvertent systemic injection, mainly in obstetric and surgical procedures, and is manifested by CNS toxicity (seizures) and a "hyper" state. This is followed by a depressive period with obtundation, hypotension, and cardiorespiratory depression. Toxicity should be differentiated from the infrequent anaphylactic reaction.

lidocaine toxicity

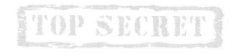

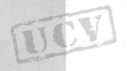

ID/CC	A 52-year-old man visits his physician complaining of **extreme tiredness, dry mouth, and easy fatigability**; he states that he has never experienced symptoms such as these before.
HPI	He was started on hydrochlorothiazide for treatment of hypertension, but it did not control his hypertension, so **α-methyldopa** was added approximately 2 months ago. On directed questioning, he states that he has been suffering from **sexual dysfunction** (impotence and inability to ejaculate) for the past several weeks.
PE	VS: BP 130/90, but when standing up it is 100/60 (ORTHOSTATIC HYPOTENSION); no fever; bradycardia (HR 58). PE: **conjunctival pallor**; oriented with regard to person, time, and place; well hydrated despite **dryness of mouth**; funduscopic exam normal; no neck masses or bruits; no lymphadenopathy; chest auscultation normal; abdomen soft and nontender with no masses; no peritoneal signs.
Labs	CBC: **positive Coombs' test**; decreased hemoglobin and hematocrit; **increased reticulocytes; decreased haptoglobin**. UA: hemoglobinuria. Increased indirect bilirubin; normal iron levels.
Imaging	CXR/KUB: normal for age.
Treatment	Switch antihypertensive treatment.
Discussion	**Methyldopa** is a **sympatholytic** that produces a false neurotransmitter, α-methyl-norepinephrine, which activates inhibitory α2-receptors in the CNS. It is used as an antihypertensive drug, and its side effects include impotence, Coombs positivity (20% of patients), and, more rarely, hemolytic anemia. It can also cause **sedation, drowsiness**, severe orthostatic hypotension, and hepatic toxicity.

methyldopa side effects

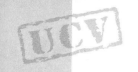
ID/CC

The 48-year-old chief executive officer of a leading auto manufacturer is put on **niacin** and a restricted diet for the treatment of **high-LDL cholesterol**.

HPI

The patient is a "bon vivant" who enjoys **drinking** and **eating** gourmet food as well as **smoking** two packs a day of Cuban filter-free dark tobacco cigarettes. On a visit two months afterward, the patient's lab tests show improvement, but he complains of **facial flushing** and **itching** on the lower back, palms, and anus.

PE

VS: mild hypertension (BP 145/95). PE: obesity; **face, neck, and chest flushed**; no skin rash demonstrable on inspection.

Labs

Serum glucose elevated (157 mg/dL); **LDL lowered** considerably in comparison to last visit; **triglycerides decreased**, but not as markedly; **HDL increased**; **AST and ALT** mildly **elevated**; **elevated uric acid**; **normal** levels of 5-hydroxyindoleacetic acid (vs. carcinoid syndrome, which may also produce facial flushing).

Imaging

CXR: normal.

Treatment

Flushing and itching are often transient. Aspirin diminishes symptoms by inhibiting prostaglandin synthesis.

Discussion

Nicotinic acid (NIACIN) is a derivative of tryptophan, a constituent of NAD and NADP that is used in redox reactions. As a drug, it is used for its lipid-lowering properties (decreases VLDL, decreases LDL, and increases HDL cholesterol). **Hepatitis, hyperglycemia,** and exacerbation of peptic ulcer are other side effects.

niacin side effects

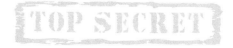

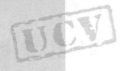
ID/CC   A 53-year-old male **chemical-factory worker** presents with **chronic headaches and dizziness** with occasional **chest pain**.

HPI   The patient states that his headaches and dizziness occur most frequently when he **returns to work** after a few days off; he is otherwise in good health.

PE   VS: mild hypertension. PE: patient appears normal but **slightly cyanotic**; neck exam shows no masses or carotid bruit; cardiac exam normal; lung fields clear; abdomen soft and nontender; no hepatosplenomegaly; no focal neurologic signs.

Labs   CBC: normal. SMA-7 normal. UA: normal. **Methemoglobin levels elevated**. ECG: no sign of ischemia or necrosis.

Imaging   CXR/KUB: within normal limits for age.

Treatment   Avoid exposure.

Discussion   Nitrates are a large class of drugs that are used in treatment of angina. All agents in this group, including nitroglycerin, act through nitric oxide (NO) release. NO, in turn, is a potent vasodilator of vascular smooth muscle. These compounds have a short half-life and may produce tolerance in chronically exposed individuals. Patients may suffer angina or MI as a result of rebound coronary vasoconstriction due to withdrawal.

nitrate exposure

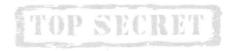

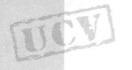

CASE 9

ID/CC

A 58-year-old man comes to see his cardiologist because of an **increased need for nitroglycerin patches** in order to control his oppressive exercise-induced chest pain (ANGINA).

HPI

In the past, taking one tablet five minutes before physical activity controlled his symptoms; now he has to take two tablets. The patient has continued to smoke two packs of cigarettes each day and is concerned that his cardiac condition is worsening because of this **increased need for medication**.

PE

VS: BP normal. PE: obese male in no acute distress; no rales or crackles on lung fields; heart sounds normal; no murmurs; no third or fourth heart sounds; fingertips cigarette-stained; no hepatosplenomegaly; no increase in JVP; no leg edema.

Labs

Elevated glucose (154 mg/dL); hypercholesterolemia; hypertriglyceridemia; BUN and creatinine normal; LFTs normal. ECG: no signs of ischemia or infarction.

Imaging

CXR: calcification of aortic knob, left ventricular hypertrophy. Echo: no segmental wall abnormalities.

Gross Pathology

Atherosclerotic narrowing of coronary arteries.

Treatment

Adjust timing of nitrate administration in order to have an 8-hour period free of nitroglycerin. Consider alternating with beta-blockers, calcium-channel-blocking agents, or other coronary vasodilators.

Discussion

Tolerance is manifested as a poor response to a previously effective dose of nitroglycerin. Increasing the dosage does not yield relief of symptoms. The use of other agents, shorter-acting nitroglycerin formulations, or intervals free of nitroglycerin dosing can be tried in an attempt to regain sensitivity to the nitrate. Tolerance and headaches are the main drawbacks of nitrate use for the treatment of angina. Progression of coronary artery disease must always be considered with increasing nitroglycerin requirements.

nitroglycerin tolerance

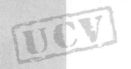

CASE 10

ID/CC
A 56-year-old male comes to the cardiology unit for evaluation of ring ing in his ears (TINNITUS), dizziness, GI distress (nausea, vomiting, and diarrhea), and headaches.

HPI
He also complains of blurred vision and impaired hearing. The patient had an MI 1 year ago and has been receiving oral quinidine antiarrhythmic therapy.

PE
VS: bradycardia (HR 55); BP normal (BP 110/70). PE: funduscopic exam normal but accommodation impaired; skin flushed; hands show fine tremors; no heart murmurs; lungs clear; abdomen soft and nontender with no masses; no peritoneal signs.

Labs
CBC: normal. Lytes: normal. ECG: prolonged Q-T interval.

Imaging
CXR: no pulmonary edema.

Treatment
Monitor ECG and vital signs; change to different antiarrhythmic drug. Treat cardiotoxic effects with sodium lactate.

Discussion
Quinidine, procainamide, and disopyramide are class IA antiarrhythmic that act by **blocking sodium channels, increasing the effective refractory period**. They are used for both atrial and ventricular arrhythmias. All these agents have low therapeutic-toxic ratios and may produce severe adverse reactions. Cinchonism is commonly produced by drug that are cinchona derivatives, such as quinidine and quinine. The effect may occur with only one dose.

quinidine side effects

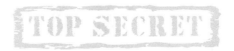

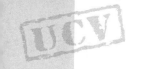

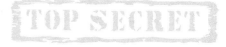

ID/CC

A 73-year-old white widow visits her cardiologist complaining of **difficulty moving her bowels** for the past week; she also reports **facial flushing**.

HPI

She had been regular until she began taking **verapamil** for an irregular heart beat 1 month ago.

PE

VS: heart rate normal; BP normal; no fever. PE: in no acute distress; no pallor; left eye cataract; no neck masses; no lymphadenopathy; lungs clear; cardiac exam normal; abdomen soft and nondistended; no palpable masses; no peritoneal signs; mild lower leg **edema**.

Labs

CBC/Lytes/UA: normal. BUN, glucose, LFTs normal; no hypercalcemia (may produce constipation); normal levels of 5-hydroxyindoleacetic acid (vs. carcinoid syndrome, which may also produce facial flushing but not constipation).

Imaging

CXR: within normal limits for age. KUB: moderate amount of stool; no sign of obstruction.

Treatment

Increase fluids in diet, regular exercise, fruits, high-bulk foods, or bulk laxatives. If persistent, change to another calcium channel blocker.

Discussion

Verapamil is one of the agents that block voltage-dependent calcium channels, consequently reducing muscle contractility. Verapamil acts more specifically on myocardial fibers than on arteriolar smooth muscle. It is widely used as an antihypertensive, as an antiarrhythmic agent, and for treatment of angina pectoris. Constipation is a common side effect; other side effects include dizziness, facial flushing, hyperprolactinemia, and peripheral edema.

verapamil side effects

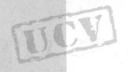
ID/CC　　A 19-year-old female is admitted to the internal medicine ward because of **generalized desquamation** of the skin, high **fever**, and painful **ulcers and bullae in her eyes and vagina**.

HPI　　She adds that **swallowing** is extremely **painful**. For the past week, she has been on oral **sulfonamides** for a urinary tract infection.

PE　　VS: fever (39.2°C). PE: painful **mucosal ulcerations** in conjunctiva, nose, mouth, oropharynx, and vagina; eyelids swollen and erythematous; **generalized, symmetric rash** on skin with **macules, papules, vesicles, and bullae** (multiple primary skin lesions) as well as areas of denudation (epidermis completely separated from dermis) on palms, soles, and extremities.

Gross Pathology　　Biopsy distinguishes from toxic epidermal necrolysis, pemphigus, and pemphigoid.

Micro Pathology　　Dermal edema with perivascular inflammatory infiltrate and epidermal separation in bullae showing necrotic and hemorrhagic areas.

Treatment　　Hospitalization, discontinue sulfa drug, prophylactic antibiotics (due to increased risk of infections acquired through large areas of denuded skin), barrier nursing, antihistamines. Steroids have not been demonstrated to be effective.

Discussion　　Also called **erythema multiforme major**, Stevens–Johnson syndrome is a grave, acute, and sometimes fatal disease with generalized skin **desquamation** and severe **ulcers and bullae** on at least two mucosal surfaces, including the genitalia, mouth, conjunctiva, nose, or lips. The use of sulfa drugs (bacteriostatic antibiotics, which are PABA antimetabolites that inhibit dihydropteroate synthase) is a common precipitating factor. Other drugs implicated are **phenytoin**, penicillins, and barbiturates.

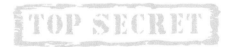

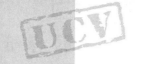

CASE 13

ID/CC A 26-year-old obsessive-compulsive female comes to the family medicine clinic to have her 5-year-old daughter checked by a dermatologist because of **itching and scaling of her skin.**

HPI The mother is very thin and fears that her daughter will not gain enough weight, so she has given her **cod-liver oil** (rich in vitamin A) **four times a day for the past nine months.** The child complains of **fatigue, headaches,** and **bone pain.**

PE Funduscopic exam reveals **papilledema** (pseudotumor cerebri); localized areas of hair loss (ALOPECIA); very **dry skin** with **scaling** areas on back and extremities; **hyperkeratosis** on medial side of soles of feet; **liver** moderately **enlarged** but not painful.

Labs Increased levels of vitamin A in serum.

Imaging XR, long bones and spine: **cortical hyperostosis; demineralization; premature closure of epiphyses.**

Treatment Discontinue administration of vitamin A-containing supplement.

Discussion Together with vitamins D, E, and K, vitamin A is one of the fat-soluble vitamins, which means that the body stores them and does not eliminate them as quickly as it does water-soluble vitamins. Vitamin A (RETINOL) is derived from carotenes and is a constituent of retinal pigments (RHODOPSIN). Vitamin A is necessary for the integrity of all epithelial cells. **Deficiency of vitamin A** produces **night blindness** and **xerophthalmia.** Vitamin A is mainly found in meat, liver, fish, and dairy products.

DERMATOLOGY

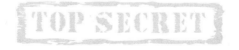

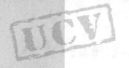

CASE 14

ID/CC   A 32-year-old male who works as a professional weight lifter comes to the family medicine clinic for evaluation of **impotence** for the past 4 months.

HPI   His girlfriend reports increasingly **aggressive** and **labile behavior**. He has a history of multiple cycles of oral and injectable **anabolic steroid abuse**.

PE   VS: **borderline hypertension**. PE: young, muscular male; androgenic **alopecia**; **acne**; **gynecomastia**; **testicular atrophy**.

Labs   CBC/Lytes: normal. AST and ALT normal; **hyperglycemia** (145 mg/dL); BUN and creatinine normal; decreased HDL; increased LDL; **oligospermia** on semen analysis.

Imaging   CXR: normal. XR, long bones and spine: normal calcification.

Treatment   Discontinue androgens.

Discussion   Anabolic steroids are widely abused by weight lifters, other athletes, and the lay public. Although androgens increase muscle mass significantly, they produce only slight increases in strength. Numerous side effects have been reported, including **hepatic neoplasia, glucose intolerance, decreased HDL-C levels, hypertension, testicular atrophy and oligospermia, virilization and amenorrhea, acne**, and **alopecia**. Other consequences of androgen abuse include mood disturbances and **irritability** that may result in **aggressive behavior** and injury to others.

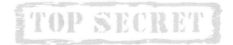

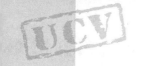
ID/CC

A 46-year-old female comes to the medical clinic for an evaluation of **weight gain, roundness of her face**, and epigastric pain that is relieved by eating (peptic ulcer).

HPI

She had been suffering from chronic, itchy blisters in the mouth that came and went, leaving painful ulcers together with large bullae on all four extremities and on her chest and lower back (PEMPHIGUS), for which she has been taking **high-dose prednisone** for several months.

PE

VS: **hypertension** (BP 145/95); no fever. PE: **moon facies, acne, buffalo hump, truncal obesity, striae, increased facial hair** (HIRSUTISM), and **ecchymoses** on distal extremities.

Labs

CBC: leukocytosis with **lymphopenia. Hyperglycemia.** Lytes: **hypokalemia.** UA: glycosuria.

Imaging

XR, spine and long bones: generalized **osteoporosis**.

Treatment

Institute steroid-sparing agents such as methotrexate, azathioprine, dapsone, or nicotinamide. Corticosteroids should be tapered down.

Discussion

Of the causes of Cushing's syndrome, iatrogenesis is the most common. Steroids produce a lysosomal membrane stabilization, blocking leukotriene formation from arachidonic acid, blocking the action of phospholipase A, and inhibiting cyclooxygenase activity (decreased prostaglandin formation). Because of this, steroids are used in a number of settings, such as acute inflammation, anaphylaxis, allergy states, and immune suppression as well as for the treatment of Addison's disease.

ENDOCRINOLOGY

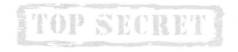

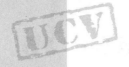

ID/CC A 32-year-old woman comes for her first gynecologic visit.

HPI On routine pelvic exam a vaginal **mass** is felt. The **patient's mother took an estrogen compound** (DES) during pregnancy as treatment for threatened abortion.

PE Well developed with breast tissue appropriate to age; pubic and axillary hair normal; on bimanual pelvic examination a **hard, ulcerated mass** is felt on posterior **wall of upper vagina**; iodine staining of vaginal wall shows patches of decreased uptake by cells (due to adenosis).

Labs CBC/Lytes/UA: normal. Hormonal screen and LFTs do not disclose any abnormality.

Imaging Hysterosalpingogram: injection of contrast into uterine cavity reveals T-shaped uterus and cervical incompetence.

Micro Pathology Biopsy by colposcopy shows glandular epithelium in upper part of vagina with squamous metaplasia (ADENOSIS). Biopsy of the ulcerated mass shows **clear-cell adenocarcinoma of vagina**.

Treatment Surgery; radiation.

Discussion Diethylstilbestrol is a synthetic estrogen that was used some 30 to 35 years ago for the prevention of a threatened abortion. The daughters of patients thus treated before the 18th week of pregnancy may present with an alteration in the development of the embryonic transition between the urogenital canal and paramesonephric system, producing persistence of the müllerian glands on the upper vagina and giving rise to adenosis and clear cell adenocarcinoma that is usually asymptomatic and discovered incidentally. Other side effects include transverse vaginal septum, developmental uterine abnormalities, and cervical incompetence. In males DES may be associated with genital tract abnormalities.

TOP SECRET

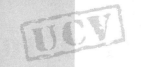

CASE 17

ID/CC

A 17-year-old white female student who is learning how to inject herself with **insulin** is found **unconscious** by her desk.

HPI

The patient suffered from weight loss, polyuria, polydipsia, and polyphagia for several months and was recently diagnosed with **juvenile-onset diabetes mellitus**. She has been meticulous in self-administering insulin injections but often injects larger doses of insulin than prescribed (over-dosing is common at the beginning of treatment).

PE

VS: **tachycardia** (HR 96); **hypotension** (BP 100/50); no fever. PE: **skin cold and moist**; patient **stuporous** with hyporeflexia; negative Babinski's sign; responsive only to painful stimuli; cardiopulmonary exam normal; no hepatomegaly; no splenomegaly; no peritoneal signs.

Labs

Severe hypoglycemia. Lytes: potassium and magnesium levels sharply decreased (HYPOKALEMIA, HYPOMAGNESEMIA). BUN and creatinine normal; increased serum levels of insulin with normal C-peptide levels.

Imaging

CT, head: no intracranial pathology demonstrated to account for the stuporous state.

Treatment

Administer IV 50% glucose or IM glucagon after drawing baseline blood sample. Follow serum glucose levels for several hours; monitor and treat electrolyte imbalances.

Discussion

With the administration of insulin, blood glucose levels are lowered by direct stimulation of cellular uptake. Glucose uptake is accompanied by a shift of magnesium and potassium into the cell. A severe hypoglycemic coma may result from an insulin overdose, which can produce **permanent neurologic damage or death**.

ENDOCRINOLOGY

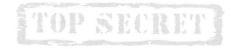

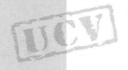

CASE 18

ID/CC A 36-year-old female oboe player is brought by ambulance to the emergency room because of gradual numbness and **weakness on the left side of her face and arm** along with **headache** and dizziness.

HPI She is **obese** and **smokes** one pack of cigarettes a day. She is currently taking **oral contraceptive pills (OCPs)**.

PE VS: normal. PE: patient conscious, oriented, and able to speak; **gaze is deviated to the right**; funduscopic exam does not show papilledema, hypertension, or diabetic retinopathy; lungs clear; abdomen soft and nontender; no peritoneal signs; **left arm and leg weakness with hyporeflexia.**

Labs CBC/Lytes: normal. **Hyperlipidemia**; BUN and creatinine normal; RPR negative; protein C and protein S negative. ECG: normal.

Imaging CT, head: negative. Arteriography: thrombotic cerebral arterial occlusion.

Treatment Intensive care treatment and surveillance for stroke in evolution. Evaluate anticoagulation, discontinue OCPs.

Discussion Oral contraceptive pills are a very popular method of birth control. There are many OCP preparations; most consist of a combination of estrogens and progestins which, when taken daily, selectively inhibit pituitary function to prevent ovulation. The most severe complication is an **increased incidence of vascular thrombotic events**, either cerebral or myocardial. Other side effects include nausea, acne, weight gain, psychological depression, cholestatic jaundice, increased incidence of vaginal infections, headaches, and breakthrough bleeding. OCPs should be used cautiously in patients with asthma, diabetes, liver disease, and hypertension.

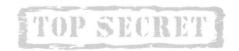

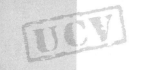

CASE 19

ID/CC A 55-year-old, **postmenopausal** white **female** complains of **nausea, headaches, weight gain, and breast tenderness**.

HPI She was placed on **estrogen** 6 months ago and is also taking **calcium** and **vitamin D**. She had a **hysterectomy** 5 years ago. There is no history of breast, uterine, or ovarian cancer in her family.

PE VS: normal. PE: mild tenderness to palpation over lumbar vertebrae; breast exam reveals diffuse tenderness without any palpable masses; no axillary lymphadenopathy.

Labs Lipid profile reveals decreased LDL, increased HDL, and elevated triglycerides.

Imaging DEXA: **osteopenia** in thoracolumbar vertebral bodies.

Treatment Discontinue estrogens and strongly consider use of nonhormonal agents (e.g., bisphosphonates, calcitonin) for long-term osteoporosis prophylaxis.

Discussion Until recently, estrogen replacement therapy (ERT) was considered to be first-line therapy for postmenopausal osteoporosis prophylaxis. In patients with an intact uterus, hormone replacement therapy (HRT) included progesterone to reduce the risk of endometrial cancer. Results from the Women's Health Initiative (WHI) trial confirmed risk reduction of osteoporotic fractures in women on ERT or HRT but found an increased risk for stroke and pulmonary embolism (ERT) as well as coronary artery disease and breast cancer (HRT). Current guidelines are evolving but tend to encourage nonhormonal treatment for the prevention of chronic disease, including osteoporosis.

ENDOCRINOLOGY

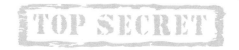

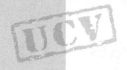

CASE 20

ID/CC	A 53-year-old, postmenopausal white female presents to the outpatient clinic with questions regarding "that bone disease" and requests a bone density scan.
HPI	She drinks at least three cups of **coffee and smokes** a pack of cigarettes daily. She is married with two children. There is no history of **alcohol** abuse, corticosteroid use, or osteoporosis among immediate family members. She **strongly refuses any oral prophylactic hormone therapy**.
PE	VS: normal. PE: unremarkable.
Imaging	DEXA: mild **osteopenia**.
Treatment	**Calcium** and **vitamin D** supplementation; regular **exercise and a balanced diet**; counsel on **fall prevention** and **smoking cessation**; alternative therapy with **bisphosphonates**, selective estrogen receptor modulators (**SERMs**), and **calcitonin**.
Discussion	Osteoporosis is a bone disease characterized by a decrease in bone density. It is classically a disease of **elderly, thin, postmenopausal Caucasian** or **Asian females** and commonly causes hip and vertebral fractures. Hip fractures can occur secondary to a **fall** but also result from repetitive stress on the hip during intensive exercise programs. **Smoking** increases the risk of osteoporosis, but **caffeine** intake is now believed to have minor or no effect on bone density or fractures. Low to moderate intake of **alcohol** is beneficial, as it increases estrogen levels. **Multiparity** is protective. Calcium is believed to **decrease bone resorption**, probably by inhibiting PTH secretion, but is far less potent than **estrogen** in preventing osteoporosis. Metabolites of **vitamin D** increase the intestinal absorption of calcium, and the most active metabolite, **calcitriol**, or $(1,25)$ OH_2 vitamin D, stimulates bone formation via osteoblasts.

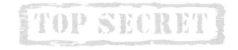

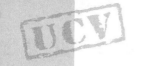

CASE 21

ID/CC

A 67-year-old, **postmenopausal white female** presents with **weakness, muscular twitching,** and a nagging **retrosternal heartburn.**

HPI

She was placed on **estrogen** and **alendronate therapy** 6 months ago following the diagnosis of a **spinal compression fracture** secondary to advanced osteoporosis. She is **not on** any **calcium or vitamin D supplementation.**

PE

VS: normal. PE: carpopedal spasm noted on inflating BP cuff (TROUSSEAU'S SIGN); facial twitching noted on tapping anterior to the tragus (CHOVSTEK'S SIGN); spinal kyphosis and protuberant abdomen.

Labs

Lytes: **hypocalcemia. Elevated PTH levels.**

Treatment

Calcium replacement with vitamin D; advise patient to **take alendronate in upright posture** to reduce reflux and risk of esophagitis; H$_2$ blockers or proton pump inhibitors for concomitant or exacerbated peptic ulcer disease/GERD.

Discussion

Bisphosphonates such as **alendronate** and **pamidronate** increase bone mass by decreasing bone resorption. Side effects include **hypocalcemia, increased PTH levels,** and **upper GI irritation/esophageal ulceration** when given orally. Other medications given for osteoporosis include **raloxifene,** a **selective estrogen receptor modulator (SERM),** and **calcitonin. Calcitonin** causes increases in bone density (not as much as seen with bisphosphonates) and is a safe alternative to estrogen. Side effects include nasal irritation when administered as a nasal spray.

ENDOCRINOLOGY

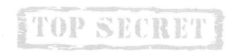

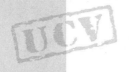

CASE 22

ID/CC	A 50-year-old white male presents with decreased libido, progressive impotence, fatigue, and muscle weakness.
HPI	He underwent a **transsphenoidal hypophysectomy** for a **large pituitary tumor** 2 months ago. He is currently on hormone replacement therapy with thyroxine and corticosteroids.
PE	VS: normal. PE: bilateral **breast enlargement** (GYNECOMASTIA), **bilateral testicular atrophy**, and **loss of facial and pubic hair**.
Labs	Decreased serum testosterone level; decreased serum LH and FSH.
Treatment	**Testosterone replacement** via either a transdermal testosterone or IM injections; long-term use of testosterone produces subjective improvement in mood, energy, libido, muscle mass, and sexual function.
Discussion	**Hypogonadism** or **testosterone deficiency** is either congenital or acquired. Causes are categorized as either **primary** (hypergonadotropic, high FSH/LH levels) or **secondary** (hypogonadotropic, low FSH/LH levels). The most common congenital cause of primary hypogonadism is Klinefelter's syndrome. Acquired causes include trauma, surgery, testicular torsion, irradiation, chemotherapy, alcoholism, and aging. Secondary hypogonadism is associated with disorders such as Kallmann's and Prader–Willi syndromes or with pituitary tumors or trauma. Side effects of testosterone include **itching** and **local irritation** (when given topically) and **liver dysfunction** and a **decrease in HDL** (when given orally). Testosterone is contraindicated in men with prostatic carcinoma.

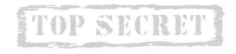

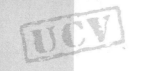

ID/CC   A **37-year-old obese male** presents with recent worsening of his anginal symptoms.

HPI   He suffers from **coronary artery disease** and regularly takes anti-anginal medications. One month ago, he began to take **Metabolife 356** for weight loss and to "increase his energy level." He drinks **three cups of coffee a day**.

PE   VS: borderline **hypertension** (BP 150/100). PE: unremarkable.

Labs   ECG: normal.

Imaging   CXR: normal.

Treatment   **Stop ephedrine** containing supplement and educate on risks of unsupervised use of herbal/alternative medicines; evaluate for worsening coronary artery disease if symptoms do not abate after stopping the supplement.

Discussion   **Herbal supplements** as alternative medicines are currently in widespread use. Over 20% of the general population use herbal supplements for health, but fewer than 50% of those taking supplements tell their physician. **Metabolife 356** is a combination of many active herbs that is sold over the counter as a weight-loss supplement. One of the ingredients in Metabolife 356 is **ephedrine (Ma Huang)**, a sympathomimetic drug that stimulates the sympathetic nervous system and is synergistic with **caffeine**. The adverse effects of ephedrine include **increased blood pressure, palpitations, chest pain, psychosis, tremor, insomnia, dry mouth**, and **cardiomyopathy** linked to chronic use.

GASTROENTEROLOGY

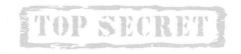

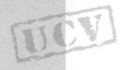

CASE 24

ID/CC A 36-year-old white morbidly obese woman presents to her primary care physician, seeking help with losing weight.

HPI She has tried various diets and exercise programs with no success.

PE VS: normal. PE: morbidly obese.

Labs CBC/Lytes: normal. Lipid panel, LFTs, TSH normal.

Treatment Orlistat or sibutramine in combination with a structured diet and exercise program.

Discussion Obesity contributes to **atherosclerosis, CAD, hyperlipidemia, hypertension, and type II diabetes**. Anti-obesity drugs currently on the market include **orlistat** and **sibutramine**. They are indicated for weight loss and maintenance in conjunction with a calorie-reduced diet in patients with a body mass index ≥ 30. Orlistat is a **lipase inhibitor** that acts in the GI tract and **blocks the absorption of dietary fat**. The most common adverse effects are GI-related and include spotting, flatus, and fatty stools. Absorption of lipid-soluble vitamins (e.g., vitamin K) or medications (e.g., griseofulvin) may be decreased. Sibutramine treats obesity through **appetite suppression**; it acts centrally by blocking serotonin and norepinephrine reuptake. Adverse effects include headache, dry mouth, constipation, insomnia, and a **substantial increase in blood pressure and heart rate in some patients**. Unlike the discontinued drug fenfluramine, sibutramine does not cause pulmonary hypertension or cardiac valve dysfunction. Sibutramine is contraindicated in patients on MAO inhibitors or SSRIs (may precipitate **serotonin syndrome**), in those with CHF/CAD, and in those with hepatic dysfunction (the drug is metabolized by **cytochrome P450**).

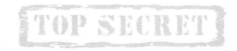

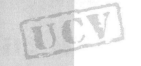
ID/CC

A 64-year-old male with **metastatic lung cancer** is seen with complaints of **severe bone pain, anorexia,** and **cachexia.**

HPI

He spends most of his time in bed because of profound weakness and chronic nausea.

PE

VS: **mild fever** (38.0°C); **tachycardia** (HR 110); **underweight** (45 kg, body mass index 17). PE: **cachetic; sunken eyes; prominent skin wrinkles/folds; visible loss of significant skeletal muscle mass.**

Labs

CBC: lymphopenia. Lytes: **hypokalemia; hypochloremia.** ABGs: **metabolic alkalosis. Decreased albumin and prealbumin/transthyretin.**

Treatment

Treat with **megestrol acetate or dronabinol** to increase appetite; adequate palliative pain medications.

Discussion

Cachexia/anorexia syndrome is characterized by progressive weight loss, lipolysis, loss of muscle mass, anorexia, diarrhea, and fever in patients with end-stage cancer or AIDS. Some drugs that have proven effective in improving appetite and treating cachexia include **megestrol acetate** and **dronabinol.** Megestrol is a synthetic progesterone that stimulates the appetite, resulting in weight gain and recovery of muscle mass. It is relatively nontoxic. Side effects are rare and include **altered menses with unpredictable bleeding** and **mild edema.** Dronabinol, a synthetic **tetrahydrocannabinol (THC),** is the active component in **marijuana** and is used to treat nausea and vomiting associated with cancer chemotherapy as well as to stimulate appetite. Side effects are due mainly to the psychoactive effects of the drug and include dizziness, ataxia, hallucinations/psychosis, tachycardia, hypertension, and URI symptoms.

GASTROENTEROLOGY

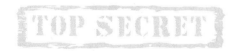

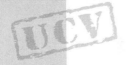

CASE 26

ID/CC	A 39-year-old male presents to his family doctor because of increasing embarrassment and concern over **breast enlargement**.
HPI	The patient has a long history of burning epigastric pain on awakening in the mornings and between meals that decreases with food and antacids (peptic ulcer disease), for which he has been taking **cimetidine**. Directed questioning reveals that he has also been suffering from **impotence**.
PE	VS: normal. PE: cardiovascular, neurologic, and abdominal examination fail to reveal any pathology; moderate bilateral growth of breast tissue; **testes** somewhat **hypotrophic**; rectal exam negative for prostatic enlargement.
Labs	CBC/Lytes/UA: normal.
Imaging	CXR/KUB: normal.
Treatment	Switch to other histamine receptor antagonists, such as ranitidine or famotidine.
Discussion	All the H_2 blockers are well tolerated, although cimetidine is associated with several side effects, particularly **reversible gynecomastia**. H_2 blockers produce an **increase in serum prolactin levels** (especially ranitidine) and alter estrogen metabolism in men (have anti-androgenic properties). Other side effects include headache, confusion, low sperm counts, and hematologic abnormalities (thrombocytopenia may enhance hypoprothrombinemic effect of oral anticoagulants). They have been largely supplanted by newer H_2 receptor blockers without many of these side effects.

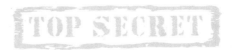

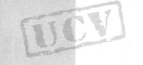

CASE 27

ID/CC

A 58-year-old female comes to the emergency room because of acute, burning **epigastric pain** accompanied by nausea and **vomiting** of **bright red blood**.

HPI

She is a chronic sufferer of rheumatoid arthritis and has taken 650 mg of **aspirin** every 8 hours for the past 4 years to control her pain.

PE

VS: **tachycardia** (HR 98); hypotension (BP 110/60); no fever. PE: **pallor**; anxiety; abdomen shows **tenderness on deep palpation in epigastrium**; no rigidity, guarding, or rebound tenderness; no masses palpable; no focal neurologic signs; hands show characteristic rheumatoid characteristics.

Labs

CBC: low hemoglobin and hematocrit. ABGs/Lytes: mild metabolic alkalosis with hypokalemia (due to vomiting of hydrochloric acid).

Imaging

Endoscopy: gastric mucosa markedly hyperemic with hemorrhagic spotting and zones of recent hemorrhage; no ulcer or tumor observed.

Treatment

Discontinue offending agent (salicylates); give prostaglandins such as **misoprostol** that inhibit acid secretion and enhance mucosal defense; replace nonselective NSAID agents with **selective cyclooxygenase inhibitors** that spare the gastric receptors, such as celecoxib; start mucosal protectors, antacids, **proton pump inhibitors**, or H_2 receptor blockers.

Discussion

Hemorrhagic gastritis is seen in individuals who take drugs that may cause damage to gastric mucosa, such as aspirin, NSAIDs, steroids, and alcohol. Critically ill patients, such as those with burns, sepsis, cranial trauma, and coagulation defects, may also bleed from the stomach. Acetylsalicylic acid (aspirin) acetylates and irreversibly inhibits cyclooxygenase 1 and 2 to prevent conversion of arachidonic acid to prostaglandins.

GASTROENTEROLOGY

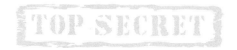

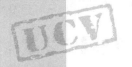

CASE 28

ID/CC   A 64-year-old female is brought to the emergency room because of the development of high fever, **marked jaundice**, weakness, profound fatigue, and **darkening of her urine**.

HPI   She has undergone many surgical procedures **under general anesthesia** (halothane) over the past 2 years, including a colpoperineoplasty, an endometrial biopsy, a femoral hernia repair, and, 4 weeks ago, a total hip replacement. After each surgery, the patient developed a low-grade fever within a few days.

PE   VS: **tachycardia** (HR 93); **hypotension** (BP 100/55); fever (39.2°C). PE: **marked weakness**; diaphoresis; patient appears **toxic**; profound **jaundice**; liver edge palpable 3 cm below costal margin and tender.

Labs   CBC: marked **leukocytosis** (18,500) with **eosinophilia** (18%) (allergic reaction). Hypoglycemia; **AST and ALT markedly elevated; elevated alkaline phosphatase and bilirubin**.

Gross Pathology   Massive centrolobular hepatic necrosis with fatty change.

Treatment   Monitor liver function; assess bilirubin, glucose levels, and PT. Provide intensive supportive care for possible hepatic failure and encephalopathy. Treat hypoglycemia with glucose, treat bleeding with fresh frozen plasma, and use lactulose to prevent encephalopathy.

Discussion   All inhaled anesthetics cause a decrease in hepatic blood flow, but rarely does this result in permanent derangement of liver function tests. Nonetheless, hydrocarbon drugs that include halothane are considered hepatotoxic. Most commonly, such drugs produce elevated LFTs, but they may also cause postoperative jaundice and hepatitis. Rarely does fulminant hepatic failure result, but such failure carries a 50% mortality rate. Occurrence is normally 4 to 6 weeks after halothane exposure. Middle-aged, obese women with several halothane exposures within closely spaced intervals are most at risk.

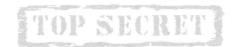

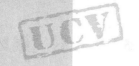

CASE 29

ID/CC

A 52-year-old HIV-positive male who was diagnosed with **tuberculosis** and started on **isoniazid** (INH) therapy 8 months ago presents with **jaundice**.

HPI

The patient's isoniazid therapy was uneventful until 2 weeks ago, when he began to appear jaundiced. He also complains of **lack of strength and sensation in his feet**.

PE

VS: normal. PE: patient appears lethargic; yellowed sclera and discoloration of skin; funduscopic exam normal; moderate, nontender hepatomegaly; decreased strength and diminished perception of light touch in feet.

Labs

Moderately **increased AST, ALT**, and **bilirubin**.

Imaging

US: generalized mild enlargement of liver with no focal lesions.

Treatment

More than a two- to threefold increase in AST and ALT warrants cessation of INH use. Also stop rifampin if it is part of multidrug therapy for tuberculosis. Substitution with second-line antitubercular agents (e.g., fluoroquinolones, aminoglycosides) may be required. Mild derangement of liver function warrants close monitoring while treatment with INH is continued. Coadministration of pyridoxine with INH is recommended to prevent and possibly ameliorate peripheral neurotoxicity.

Discussion

Isoniazid (isonicotinic acid hydrazide) decreases the synthesis of mycolic acids and is the bactericidal drug of choice for tuberculosis prophylaxis. It is used as combination therapy for eradication of *Mycobacterium tuberculosis*. Chronic use is associated with **hepatitis, peripheral neuritis,** disulfiram-like reaction, and **systemic lupus erythematosus**. INH competes with pyridoxine for the enzyme apotryptophanase, thus producing a deficiency of pyridoxine. The administration of pyridoxine can prevent some central and peripheral nervous system effects. The risk for hepatitis and multilobular necrosis is greater in alcoholics and older persons.

GASTROENTEROLOGY

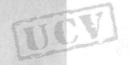
ID/CC   A 22-year-old female presents to the ER with severe abdominal colic and a history of **profuse watery diarrhea** of several days' duration.

HPI   She also complains of **dizziness** and a **desire to lose weight** (directed questioning discloses that she has been taking **magnesium sulfate** intermittently).

PE   VS: **hypotension** (BP 80/45); no fever. PE: **skin shriveled; bowel sounds hyperactive**; oliguric and lethargic.

Labs   Lytes: hypokalemia; hyponatremia; hyperchloremia. ABGs: normal anion gap metabolic acidosis.

Treatment   Discontinue laxatives and offer counseling; electrolyte and fluid replacement.

Discussion   Laxative abuse remains a common way people attempt to lose weight; abuse is also common among psychiatric patients. Laxatives can interfere with the absorption of several medications, such as tetracycline and calcium supplements. Laxatives may act by irritating the mucosa, through direct neuronal stimulation, via an osmotic increase in the water content of stool, through softening of stool by a detergent-like action, or by forming bulk. Continued abuse may lead to melanosis coli, colonic neuronal degeneration, and the "lazy intestine syndrome." Patients with chronic constipation abuse laxatives to the point of being dependent on them for evacuation.

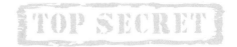

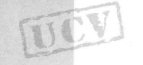

CASE 31

ID/CC

A 28-year-old white female has surgery due to perforated appendicitis with peritonitis; 10 days postoperatively she develops fever, abdominal cramping, and **diarrhea with pus and mucus**.

HPI

Her postoperative recovery was unremarkable until the onset of diarrhea. She had **received continuous parenteral antibiotics (clindamycin)**.

PE

VS: fever; tachycardia; tachypnea. PE: moderate dehydration; mild abdominal tenderness with no signs of peritoneal irritation; surgical wound normal.

Labs

CBC: leukocytosis. Stool culture reveals gram-positive rods, *Clostridium difficile*; **presence of toxin in stool**.

Imaging

Sigmoidoscopy: mucosal hyperemia, ulcers, and **pseudomembranes**.

Gross Pathology

Mucosa hyperemic and swollen; epithelial ulcerations covered by yellowish plaques (pseudomembranes) and fibrinous exudate.

Micro Pathology

Fibrinous exudate with pseudomembrane formation; ulceration of superficial epithelium; neutrophilic infiltrate with necrotic debris.

Treatment

Cessation of offending antibiotic; give **metronidazole** or oral vancomycin.

Discussion

Pseudomembranous colitis is defined as acute inflammation of the colon in patients taking antibiotics, specifically **clindamycin** or ampicillin, due to **overgrowth of *C. difficile***; it is characterized by formation of **pseudomembranes**. Clindamycin acts by blocking protein synthesis at the 50S ribosomal unit. Its main clinical indication is for life-threatening infections with **anaerobes**.

GASTROENTEROLOGY

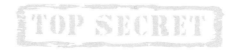

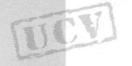

CASE 32

ID/CC	A 6-year-old boy is brought by his parents to the emergency room in a **comatose state**.
HPI	The child had been suffering from **chickenpox** and had been given **aspirin** by the family physician for fever.
PE	VS: **fever**. PE: comatose child with **papulovesicular rash** all over body; fundus shows **marked papilledema**; no icterus; moderate hepatomegaly; asterixis.
Labs	Marked hypoglycemia; increased blood ammonia concentration; elevated AST and ALT; prolonged PT; serum bilirubin normal. LP (done after lowering raised intracranial pressure): normal CSF.
Imaging	CT: findings suggestive of **generalized cerebral edema**.
Gross Pathology	Severe cerebral edema; acute hepatic necrosis.
Micro Pathology	Liver biopsy reveals microvesicular steatosis with little or no inflammation; electron microscopy shows marked mitochondrial abnormalities.
Treatment	Specific therapy not available. Supportive measures include lactulose to control hyperammonemia, fresh frozen plasma to replenish clotting factors, mannitol or dexamethasone to lower increased intracranial pressure, and mechanical ventilation. Exchange transfusion; dialysis.
Discussion	Although the cause of the highly lethal Reye's syndrome (hepatoencephalopathy) is unknown, epidemiologic evidence strongly links this disorder with outbreaks of viral disease, especially influenza B and chickenpox. Epidemiologic evidence has also prompted the Surgeon General and the American Academy of Pediatrics Committee on Infectious Diseases to recommend that **salicylates not be given to children with chickenpox or influenza B**.

TOP SECRET

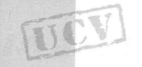

CASE 33

ID/CC

A 51-year-old chemical engineer who manages the production line at a large **petrochemical plant** comes to his family doctor for a yearly checkup; he is asymptomatic but is found to have **microscopic** painless **hematuria**.

HPI

He is a **heavy smoker** and has been working at the production plant over a period of 25 years.

PE

VS: normal. PE: strongly built male with gray hair and smoke discoloration of his mustache and fingertips; a few wheezes heard on lung fields; heart sounds normal; abdominal exam normal; no lymphadenopathy; genitalia normal; rectal exam normal.

Labs

CBC/Lytes: normal. Clinical chemistry and LFTs normal; BUN and creatinine normal. UA: **hematuria**.

Imaging

US: no renoureteral lithiasis; no pelvicalyceal dilatation. Excretory urography: filling defect and rigidity in wall of urinary bladder.

Micro Pathology

Urine cytology shows marked dysplastic and anaplastic transitional cells; cystoscopy and biopsy confirm a **papillary transitional cell carcinoma (TCC) of the bladder**.

Treatment

Surgery, chemotherapy, radiotherapy.

Discussion

The substances 2-amino-1-naphthol and p-diphenylamine are the two carcinogens that are presumed to be involved in the genesis of transitional cell bladder cancer in individuals exposed to anilines, benzidine, and β-naphthylamines. Saccharin has been shown to induce TCC in rats. Cigarette smoking greatly increases the risk. Heavy caffeine consumption remains a controversial risk factor.

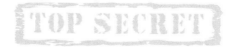

HEMATOLOGY/ONCOLOGY

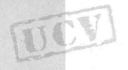

ID/CC   A **73-year-old** farmer complains of **dry cough** of 2 months' duration together with intermittent **fever, vomiting,** and increasing **dyspnea.**

HPI   He had a squamous cell carcinoma lesion surgically removed from his nose several months ago and received chemotherapy with **bleomycin.**

PE   Healed skin flap on left nasal fossa; no local lymphadenopathy; multiple freckles and solar dermatitis on scalp; scattered lung **rales and wheezing; soles of feet** show painful, erythematous areas with **skin thickening.**

Labs   CBC/Lytes: normal. LFTs normal; BUN and creatinine normal. PFTs: decreased FEV_1 and FVC with normal FEV_1/FVC ratio.

Imaging   CXR: bilateral pulmonary infiltrates but no evidence of metastatic disease.

Micro Pathology   Lung biopsy shows interstitial pneumonitis with fibrosis and bronchiolar squamous metaplasia.

Treatment   Steroids, antibiotics, discontinue bleomycin.

Discussion   Bleomycin is an antibiotic produced by *Streptomyces verticillus* that acts by DNA fragmentation. It is used in a variety of epidermoid and testicular cancers. Fever and chills may ensue with the administration of the drug by any of the parenteral routes available (it is not active orally). It has very little marrow toxicity and almost no immune suppression, but the keratinized areas of the body may suffer from hypertrophy and nail pigmentation. **Pulmonary fibrosis** is a side effect that characteristically arises in older patients and in those with preexisting lung disease.

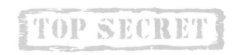

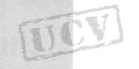

CASE 35

ID/CC   A 20-year-old male with testicular cancer presents to his oncologist with a pronounced **decrease in bilateral auditory acuity.**

HPI   His last two chemotherapy sessions were administered by an intern who only recently arrived at the municipal hospital.

PE   VS: normal. PE: auditory testing shows bilateral **neurosensory deficit in the high-frequency range**; lung fields do not show crackles or wheezing; heart sounds rhythmic with no murmurs; abdomen soft with no masses; neurologic exam reveals loss of **proprioception** in feet and diminished sensation in hands and feet (STOCKING-GLOVE PATTERN).

Labs   CBC: normal. Lytes: **hypomagnesemia; hypocalcemia**; hypernatremia; hypokalemia. **BUN and creatinine increased.**

Imaging   CT, head: no intracranial causes of hearing loss revealed.

Treatment   Vigorous hydration and diuresis to reduce severity of aeate nephrotoxicity; electrolyte replacement; pretreatment with amifostine may reduce nephrotoxicity and neurotoxicity.

Discussion   Cisplatin is an effective chemotherapeutic drug that acts like an alkylating agent, cross-linking DNA via the hydrolysis of chloride groups and reaction with platinum. It is used for bladder and testicular cancers as well as for some ovarian tumors. It can produce severe **renal damage** if administered in the absence of abundant hydration. It also causes **CN VIII damage** with permanent deafness. Another side effect is **peripheral neuropathy.**

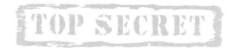

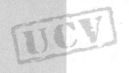

CASE 36

ID/CC   A 40-year-old male who has been diagnosed with pemphigus vulgaris complains of **dysuria** and **increased urinary frequency**.

HPI   The patient has no history of fever or gross hematuria. He is receiving monthly dexamethasone-**cyclophosphamide pulse therapy**.

PE   VS: normal. PE: no pallor; lungs clear to auscultation; cardiac exam normal; abdomen soft and nontender; no suprapubic masses; no peritoneal signs; no tenderness in costovertebral angle.

Labs   CBC: normocytic, normochromic **anemia**; mild leukopenia and thrombocytopenia. UA: **microscopic hematuria** but no bacteriuria.

Treatment   Maintain good hydration and HCO_3 loading; ε-amino caproic acid and mesna may prevent hemorrhagic cystitis.

Discussion   Cyclophosphamide is an alkylating agent that covalently cross-links DNA at guanine N-7 and requires bioactivation by the liver. It is used for lymphomas and for breast and ovarian carcinomas. Complications of cyclophosphamide use include **hemorrhagic cystitis, bladder fibrosis** and **bladder carcinoma**; sterility; alopecia; and inappropriate ADH secretion. Cyclophosphamide needs to be converted to an active toxic metabolite, **acrolein**, which is responsible for producing hemorrhagic cystitis.

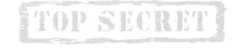

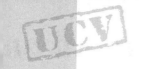
ID/CC

A 59-year-old female currently being treated for breast cancer is brought by ambulance to the ER after fainting while at work.

HPI

The patient had noticed a painless lump in her right breast 6 months earlier. She was diagnosed with invasive ductal carcinoma on biopsy and placed on an adjuvant chemotherapy regimen that included doxorubicin and cyclophosphamide.

PE

VS: **tachycardia** (HR 110); BP normal (118/85). PE: **elevated JVP**; S3 auscultated; **basal rales** in lung fields; **hepatomegaly**; **pitting edema** in lower legs.

Labs

ECG: ST-T changes, premature ventricular contractions; decreased QRS voltage.

Imaging

CXR: cardiomegaly and pulmonary congestion. Echo: dilated cardiomyopathy with reduced ejection fraction.

Gross Pathology

Increase in weight and size of heart with softened, weak walls and dilated chambers (DILATED CARDIOMYOPATHY).

Treatment

Treatment of heart failure due to **dilated cardiomyopathy**. Discontinue doxorubicin.

Discussion

Doxorubicin, also called adriamycin, is an anthracycline antibiotic that binds to DNA and blocks the synthesis of new RNA and/or DNA, thereby blocking cell replication. It is used in the treatment of carcinomas of the ovary, breast, testicle, lung, and thyroid. It is also used in the treatment of many types of sarcomas and hematologic cancers. Side effects are mainly cardiac but may also include alopecia and marrow toxicity (cardiomyopathy associated with doxorubicin is dose-related and irreversible; the mechanisms may be related to the intracellular production of free radicals in myocardium, which can be prevented by **dexrazoxane**).

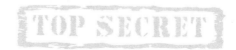

HEMATOLOGY/ONCOLOGY

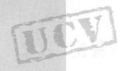

ID/CC   A 74-year-old female who recently had hip replacement surgery has been on **postoperative IV heparin** for 5 days for the prevention of possible pulmonary embolism; shortly thereafter, she starts to have black, tarry stools (MELENA, GI BLEEDING), hematuria, and **bleeding from the gums** when brushing her teeth.

HPI   She suffers from long-standing cardiac disease and has a **history of deep venous thrombosis.** However, the dose administered was excessive.

PE   VS: no fever; **heart rate slightly elevated above baseline**; BP within normal limits but drops when patient stands up (ORTHOSTATIC HYPOTENSION). PE: **pallor**; no signs of cardiac failure; **incision is oozing blood**; venipuncture sites show large **ecchymoses.**

Labs   CBC: normocytic, normochromic **anemia** (7.3 mg/dL). **aPTT and PT markedly elevated.**

Imaging   CXR: within normal limits for age. XR, hip: no evidence of hematoma formation.

Treatment   Stop heparin; for significant bleeding complications, IV **protamine sulfate** is the specific antidote.

Discussion   Heparin complexes with **antithrombin III** to form a potent **inactivator of factor Xa** and **inhibitor of the conversion of prothrombin** to thrombin. This complex also inactivates factors IXa, XIa, and XIIa. Its major adverse effect is bleeding, which occurs with a higher incidence in women over age 60. Other adverse effects include hypersensitivity, hyperlipidemia, hyperkalemia, osteoporosis, and, in up to 30% of patients, thrombocytopenia. The severity of thrombocytopenia appears to be dose related and is due to the direct effect of heparin on platelets or to an immunoglobulin that aggregates platelets.

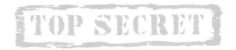

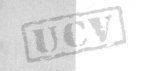

CASE 39

ID/CC

A 9-year-old male is brought to the emergency room after intentionally ingesting half a bottle of **iron tablets** (coated with plum-flavored sugar) 6 hours ago; he now complains of **abdominal pain and diarrhea**.

HPI

He has been feeling weak and lightheaded, with palpitations and a metallic taste in his mouth. He had two episodes of **bluish-green vomit** followed by a large **hematemesis**.

PE

VS: marked **tachycardia** (HR 120); **hypotension** (BP 90/50); no fever. PE: pulse weak; patient is **pale and dehydrated** with cold and clammy skin; lungs clear; abdomen tender to deep palpation, predominantly in epigastrium, with no peritoneal signs; neurologic exam normal; rectal exam discloses black, tarry stool.

Labs

Markedly elevated serum iron levels (> 500 mg/dL). UA: rose-wine-colored urine. ABGs: metabolic acidosis. BUN and creatinine elevated.

Imaging

XR, abdomen: multiple **radiopaque iron tablets** in GI tract from stomach to jejunum. Endoscopy: **diffuse hemorrhagic gastritis** with extensive necrosis and sloughing of mucosa.

Treatment

Gastric lavage with bicarbonate solution (to form ferrous carbonate, which is not absorbed well) or induction of vomiting. Treat acidosis; treat shock with IV fluids and **chelation** therapy with **deferoxamine**.

Discussion

Mortality due to acute iron overdose may reach 25% or more, mainly in children. There may be marked dehydration and shock.

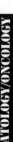

HEMATOLOGY/ONCOLOGY

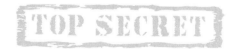

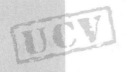

CASE 40

ID/CC   A 62-year-old female comes to the general oncology unit of the university hospital for **ulceration of the oral mucosa and diarrhea**.

HPI   She is being treated for carcinoma of the breast with aggressive methotrexate therapy.

PE   VS: hypotension (BP 100/50); tachycardia (HR 105). PE: lethargic and dehydrated; oral mucosa and tongue show erythema and shallow ulcer (BUCCAL STOMATITIS); skin rash on volar aspect of forearms.

Labs   CBC: **anemia; thrombocytopenia; leukopenia** (myelosuppression). BUN and creatinine elevated.

Treatment   The efficacy of leucovorin therapy depends on early administration when methotrexate toxicity is suspected. Give IV dose equal to or greater than the dose of methotrexate.

Discussion   Methotrexate binds **reversibly** with dihydrofolate reductase, preventing the synthesis of purine and pyrimidine nucleotides. The toxic effects of proliferating tissues are particularly deleterious to the bone marrow, skin, and GI mucosa. Leucovorin "rescue" attenuates some of these toxic effects because it is a metabolically active form of folic acid. For that reason, it does not require reduction by dihydrofolate reductase. Therefore leucovorin has the capacity to catalyze the one-carbon transfer reactions necessary for purine and pyrimidine biosynthesis.

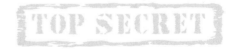

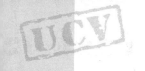
ID/CC   A 53-year-old woman presents with **dizziness and spontaneous severe bruising.**

HPI   She reports passage of several dark, tarry stools (MELENA). She underwent a valve replacement several months ago and is currently taking **warfarin** (COUMADIN) for anticoagulation prophylaxis. One week ago, she was given **co-trimoxazole** (a sulfa antibiotic) for a "sinus infection," but she neglected to tell her doctor about the Coumadin.

PE   VS: **orthostatic hypotension** (BP 110/70, HR 95 when supine; BP 90/60, HR 110 when erect). PE: extensive ecchymoses and petechiae noted on skin exam; black, tarry guaiac positive stools on rectal exam.

Labs   CBC: **anemia. PT, INR, PTT markedly elevated.**

Treatment   Supportive (blood transfusion and IV fluids); for significant bleeding complications associated with warfarin use (as in this case), withhold warfarin, administer **fresh frozen plasma** and parenteral **vitamin K**, and monitor serial PT/PTT/INR.

Discussion   **Warfarin** is an **anticoagulant** commonly used in patients with **underlying hypercoagulable states, prosthetic cardiac valves, cardiac arrhythmias, DVTs, and pulmonary embolism.** It acts by interfering with the hepatic synthesis of vitamin K-dependent clotting factors, resulting in depletion of factors VII, IX, X, and II. Warfarin is highly **protein bound**, primarily to albumin, and is metabolized by the hepatic **cytochrome P450 enzyme system. Drug interactions** with warfarin are extensive. They include increased effect due to inhibition of metabolism (e.g., amiodarone, cimetidine, co-trimoxazole), possible increased effect due to displacement from albumin (e.g., chloral hydrate, furosemide), and decreased effect due to induction of metabolism (e.g., barbiturates, rifampin).

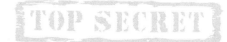

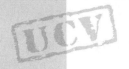

CASE 42

ID/CC	A 32-year-old male with a prosthetic heart valve complains to his family doctor of **black, tarry stools**.
HPI	He had been receiving **oral warfarin** (COUMADIN) to prevent thrombus formation. Two years ago, he had an **aortic valve replacement** due to destruction of the valve secondary to bacterial endocarditis.
PE	VS: BP normal; pulse rate normal. PE: subconjunctival hemorrhage; bleeding gums; **bruises and petechiae** on arms and legs (generalized bleeding).
Labs	Stool guaiac positive. UA: hematuria. **Markedly elevated PT** (affect extrinsic coagulation pathway).
Treatment	If significant bleeding and volume depletion have occurred, consider fresh frozen plasma and transfusions. Vitamin K may be required.
Discussion	This patient has generalized bleeding, including GI tract bleeding secondary to warfarin treatment. Warfarin compounds inhibit epoxide reductase and hepatic production of the vitamin K-dependent clotting factors (II, VII, IX, and X), interfering with their γ-carboxylation. Only de novo synthesis is affected; therefore, therapy must continue for 2 to 3 days before effects are noted. Effects of warfarin last between 5 and 7 days. Warfarin crosses the placenta and is thus contraindicated in pregnant women.

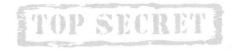

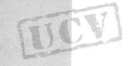

ID/CC A 45-year-old male who received a **renal transplant** 4 months ago comes to the oncology unit for a follow-up exam complaining of headache and ringing in his ears. He was found to have **hypertension**.

HPI He is currently taking multiple **immunosuppressive** drugs, including **cyclosporine**.

PE VS: **hypertension** (BP 150/110). PE: no jaundice; no pallor; cardiac exam normal; abdomen soft and nontender; no abdominal masses; no peritoneal signs; fine hand **tremors** at rest.

Labs Elevated cyclosporine levels; **elevated BUN and serum creatinine**. Lytes: **hyperkalemia**. UA: **proteinuria**. ECG: peaked T waves (hyperkalemia).

Micro Pathology Renal biopsy reveals presence of tubular lesions (vacuolization), atrophy, edema, microcalcifications, and absence of an acute cellular infiltrate that is characteristic of acute rejection.

Treatment Reduction in cyclosporine dose with serial monitoring.

Discussion Cyclosporine is an immunosuppressive agent used for the prevention of rejection in organ transplantation. Subacute nephrotoxicity is the most important side effect and is frequently seen in the first weeks or months following transplantation. Other side effects include hypertension, hyperkalemia, hyperuricemia (gout), hyperglycemia, neurotoxicity (tremor, irritability, seizure), and an increased incidence of EBV-related B-cell lymphomas. Cyclosporine is metabolized in the liver by the cytochrome P450 system.

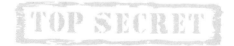

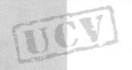
ID/CC   A 58-year-old female presents with **persistent fever, chills, headache** **weakness**, and **diffuse muscle and bone aches**.

HPI   She was diagnosed with **chronic myelocytic leukemia** (CML) a fe months ago and is now being treated with oral hydroxyurea and sut cutaneous **interferon**.

PE   VS: **fever** (39.0°C); **tachycardia** (HR 105). PE: appears fatigue splenomegaly on abdominal exam.

Labs   CBC: **anemia**; mild **leukopenia**; mild **thrombocytopenia**. No blast cel seen.

Treatment In the presence of intolerable side effects, replace interferon with alte native therapy.

Discussion Interferons are **cytokines** with antiviral, antiproliferative, and immune modulating properties. They are used to treat chronic hepatitis B, C, D infection (α2b), condyloma acuminatum (genital warts) due to HP (α2b, αn3), CML or hairy-cell leukemia (α2a, α2b), Kaposi's sarcom (α2a, α2b), melanoma (α2b), and chronic granulomatous disease (γ2b Side effects include **fever, chills, myalgias, fatigue, pancytopenia**, an **neurotoxicity** that presents as **somnolence** and **confusion**. Autoimmur phenomena, including **thyroiditis** (both hypo- and hyperthyroidism **autoimmune hemolytic anemia**, and **thrombocytopenia**, can also occu secondary to interferon use.

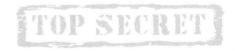

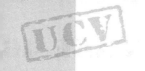

ID/CC

During ward rounds, a 28-year-old HIV-positive female patient complains that after a period of improvement since her admission 3 days ago, she now feels very sick, with **high fever**, **marked lightheadedness**, **headache**, and **myalgias**.

HPI

She was admitted because of **cryptococcal meningitis** and was started on **amphotericin B**.

PE

VS: tachycardia (HR 93); **hypotension** (BP 90/55); **fever** (39.3°C); **tachypnea**. PE: nuchal rigidity resolved; mental status improved.

Labs

CBC: mild **anemia**; normal leukocytes. Lytes: **hypokalemia**. BUN and **creatinine** moderately **elevated**.

Treatment

If the reaction is severe, it may be necessary to lower the dosage of amphotericin B, use a liposomal form, or change to fluconazole. Pretreatment with antipyretics, antihistamines, and corticosteroids may lessen febrile symptoms.

Discussion

The mechanism of action of amphotericin B is by **binding to ergosterol in fungi** and forming membrane pores. Toxicities include **arrhythmias**, **chills and fever**, **hypotension**, and **nephrotoxicity**.

INFECTIOUS DISEASE

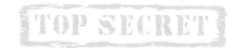

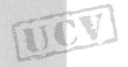

CASE 46

ID/CC   A 31-year-old truck driver visits a health clinic in San Diego complaining of **recurrent infections** (neutropenia), excessive **bleeding** (thrombocytopenia) and malaise, **weakness**, and apathy (anemia).

HPI   He travels south of the border daily and eats and sleeps there. He has had **typhoid fever** three times over the past 5 years, for which he has been treated with high-dose **chloramphenicol**.

PE   VS: no fever; BP normal. PE: marked **pallor**; lungs clear; heart sounds normal; generalized **petechiae**; abdominal and neurologic examination unremarkable.

Labs   CBC: **anemia** (Hb 5.7); **leukopenia**; **thrombocytopenia**.

Imaging   CXR/KUB: within normal limits.

Treatment   Blood transfusions, antithymocyte globulin or cyclosporin, marrow transplantation.

Discussion   Chloramphenicol is a bacteriostatic antibiotic that acts by inhibiting peptidyl transferase in the 50S ribosomal unit. It is active against anaerobes (abdominal sepsis) and rickettsiae as well as against typhoid fever and meningococcal, streptococcal, and *Haemophilus influenzae* meningitis. **Aplastic anemia** is nonetheless a major problem. Some aplastic cases appear to be related to overdose, while others are related to hypersensitivity to the drug. In infants, it produces the **gray-baby syndrome**. Owing to its potentially fatal side effect of **aplastic anemia**, chloramphenicol is used primarily for serious infections or acute *Salmonella typhi* infection.

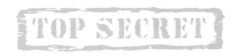

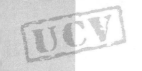

ID/CC

A 37-year-old missionary returning home from central **Africa** comes to the tropical medicine department of the local university for an evaluation of **blurred vision** and seeing "**halos**" around **lights** at night.

HPI

He also complains of marked **itching while showering** and notes that his **hair** has been turning prematurely **gray**. He has been taking **chloroquine** for the prophylaxis of hyperendemic malaria.

PE

"Half-moon-shaped" **corneal deposits** on funduscopic exam; diminished visual acuity bilaterally and **retinal edema** with pigmentation; slight **desquamation of palms of hands**; lungs clear; no heart murmurs; no hepatosplenomegaly; no focal neurologic signs.

Labs

CBC: moderate **leukopenia**.

Imaging

CXR: within normal limits.

Treatment

Discontinue chloroquine or change to mefloquine as prophylaxis.

Discussion

Chloroquine, a 4-aminoquinoline (acts by blocking DNA and RNA synthesis), is still one of the most widely used drugs for the prophylaxis and treatment of malaria, although resistant strains are becoming increasingly common. Its side effects include headache, dizziness, defects in lens accommodation with frontal heaviness, epigastralgia, diarrhea, and itching (primarily in dark-skinned people). It is also used to treat amebiasis, rheumatoid arthritis, and lupus erythematosus. When taken for long periods, it produces retinal edema with macular hyperpigmentation and chloroquine deposits with visual field defects as well as semicircular corneal opacities.

INFECTIOUS DISEASE

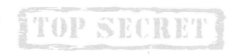

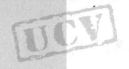

CASE 48

ID/CC	A 25-year-old male presents with **spiking fevers, malaise, left-sided chest pain**, and **cough**.
HPI	His symptoms started two weeks ago and have progressively worsened despite a full course of oral antibiotics. He also reports a history of prior **IV drug abuse**.
PE	VS: **fever** (39.2°C); **tachycardia** (HR 105); **tachypnea**. PE: "amphoric" breath sounds heard over left lower lobe; S1 and S2 normally heard without murmurs, gallops or rubs.
Labs	CBC: **leukocytosis, predominantly neutrophilic**. Blood cultures negative; induced sputum cultures grew **methicillin-resistant *Staphylococcus aureus***.
Imaging	XR, chest: 2- by 3-cm cavity in left lower lobe of lung with air-fluid level. CT, chest: confirmed a left lower lobe **lung abscess**.
Treatment	Intravenous **vancomycin** therapy; add an **aminoglycoside** for synergistic bactericidal effect.
Discussion	**Antibiotic resistance** is continuing to increase in both the hospital (nosocomial infections) and the community. Major resistant nosocomial organisms include *S. aureus*, **vancomycin-resistant enterococcus (VRE)**, *Klebsiella, Enterobacter, Escherichia coli, Pseudomonas,* and *Acinetobacter*. Multidrug-resistant bacteria causing community-acquired infections include **pneumococcus, gonococcus, *Mycobacterium tuberculosis*, group A streptococci**, and *E. coli*. Methicillin-resistant *S. aureus* (MRSA) is becoming widespread in a number of communities and is more commonly seen in **IV drug abusers, patients with recent hospitalizations**, and **residents in chronic care facilities**. Antibiotic resistance arises from numerous factors, including **colonization in hospital patients** and **frequent antibiotic use/abuse in the community**.

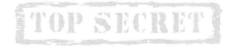

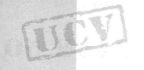
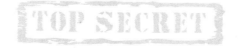

ID/CC   A 21-year-old college baseball player restarted his training 3 days ago, running 1,600 meters a day in preparation for the upcoming state tournament; yesterday he hit a home run and started off to first base when he suddenly fell to the ground and **could not walk** due to **acute pain** in the **Achilles tendon.**

HPI   He had spent 4 weeks in the hospital recovering from perforated appendicitis with peritonitis, where he received **IV ciprofloxacin** for 2 weeks due to a surgical wound infection with *Pseudomonas aeruginosa* that was resistant to all other antibiotics.

PE   Surgical wound completely healed with no evidence of infection or postincisional hernia; Penrose drain orifice within normal limits; **inability to plantarflex left foot; Achilles tendon completely severed.**

Labs   CBC: no leukocytosis; no anemia. SMA-7 normal. UA: normal.

Imaging   CXR/KUB: within normal limits.

Micro Pathology   Achilles tendon shows inflammatory neutrophilic infiltrate with areas of hemorrhage and necrosis.

Treatment   Surgical repair.

Discussion   Fluoroquinolones such as ciprofloxacin and norfloxacin are bactericidal antibiotics that are active against gram-negative rods, including *Pseudomonas*; they are also active against *Neisseria* and some gram-positive organisms. They act by **inhibiting DNA gyrase** (TOPOISOMERASE II). Side effects include **damage to cartilage** (contraindicated in pregnancy and small children), tendonitis, and tendon rupture; they also produce gastric upset and nausea and may cause superinfections.

INFECTIOUS DISEASE

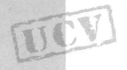

CASE 50

ID/CC A 34-year-old woman presents with her family practitioner complaining of **hearing loss, vertigo**, and inability to walk properly due to **lack of balance**.

HPI She is an otherwise healthy individual who underwent a left salpingectomy for pyosalpinx and was put on IV **gentamicin** for 10 days.

PE Well hydrated, oriented, cooperative; gait is ataxic; abdomen shows well healed, infraumbilical midline scar with no evidence of post-op hernia, infection, or hematoma.

Labs **Elevated BUN** and **serum creatinine**; fractional excretion of sodium markedly increased (> 1%). UA: **dark brown granular casts** with free renal tubular epithelial cells and epithelial cell casts. ECG: normal sinus rhythm; no conduction abnormalities or signs of ischemia.

Imaging CXR: fails to disclose any lung infection or cardiac abnormality to account for the patient's symptoms.

Treatment Supportive. Discontinuation of the aminoglycoside; resolution of acute episode may be delayed if patient remains hypovolemic, septic, or catabolic.

Discussion Gentamicin is an aminoglycoside and thus shares the ototoxicity and nephrotoxicity of streptomycin, kanamycin, amikacin, and tobramycin. Ototoxicity is mainly cochlear and marked by ataxia and vertigo. Nephrotoxicity is minimized if care is taken to hydrate the patient and keep serum levels therapeutic. Transient elevations of BUN and creatinine are common.

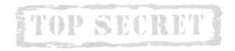

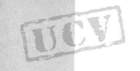

CASE 51

ID/CC A 23-year-old marathon runner visits his sports-medicine doctor complaining of unsightly, embarrassing **growth of his right breast** (GYNECOMASTIA) as well as **undue fatigue** after training and a slight yellowish hue in his eyes (JAUNDICE).

HPI Three months ago, he was put on daily oral **ketoconazole** because he had been suffering from a severe, refractory tinea corporis infection.

PE VS: bradycardia; **fever** (38.1°C). PE: slight jaundice in conjunctiva; no lymphadenopathy; no neck masses; cardiopulmonary exam normal; no hepatomegaly; examination of skin reveals tinea corporis covering intertriginous areas, buttocks, and scrotum.

Labs **AST and ALT increased**; serum bilirubin level increased.

Imaging US, liver: mildly enlarged liver.

Treatment Discontinue drug; substitute treatment with alternative antifungal (e.g., terbinafine).

Discussion Ketoconazole is an imidazole that inhibits fungal synthesis of ergosterol in membranes. It is used for blastomycosis, coccidioidomycosis, histoplasmosis, and candidiasis. Major side effects are **hepatic damage, gynecomastia, impotence** (due to inhibition of testosterone synthesis), inhibition of cytochrome P450, fever, and chills. When taken with antacids or H_2 receptor blockers, its absorption is decreased. It dramatically increases cyclosporine levels.

INFECTIOUS DISEASE

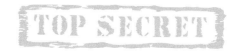

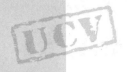

CASE 52

ID/CC   A 21-year-old male comes to the health clinic because of the development of **fever**, marked **itching** all over his body, a **generalized rash** with **joint swelling**, and **difficulty breathing**.

HPI   He just returned from a trip abroad, where he had developed a **purulent urethral discharge** (gonococcal urethritis) and went to a local doctor who gave him "two shots on each side" preceded by two pills (procain penicillin and probenecid).

PE   VS: mild **hypotension**. PE: in acute distress; mild cyanosis and difficult breathing; eyelids, lips, and tongue **edematous**; large **hives** on hands and chest.

Labs   CBC: leukocytosis (12,000 with 60% neutrophils). Lytes: normal.

Imaging   CXR: normal.

Treatment   Subcutaneous epinephrine, oxygen, hydrocortisone, antihistamines. Maintain airway and provide assisted ventilation if necessary. Sever reactions may result in laryngeal obstruction, hypotension, and death.

Discussion   Penicillins are antimicrobial drugs that block cell wall synthesis by inhibiting peptidoglycan cross-linking; they are bactericidal for gram positive cocci and rods, gram-negative cocci, and spirochetes such as *Treponema pallidum*. Most adverse reactions to penicillin are allergic reactions that result when one of its metabolites acts as a hapten. Anaphylactic (TYPE I HYPERSENSITIVITY) reaction involves antigen reacting with IgE on presensitized mast cells and basophils; it is usually severe and immediate. Penicillin may also give rise to a **serum sickness** (TYPE III HYPERSENSITIVITY) reaction, an immune complex disorder with a lag period during which antibodies are formed. This results in fever, edema, malaise, arthralgias, and arthritis.

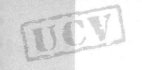

CASE 53

ID/CC

A 19-year-old military recruit comes to his medical officer complaining of **red urine** and **orange-colored staining of his T-shirt**; he also complains that every time he takes rifampin, he feels as if he has the flu (flulike response).

HPI

He underwent a routine physical exam and laboratory tests prior to joining the military camp and was started on **rifampin** at that time (meningococcus was found in nasopharyngeal secretions, indicating a meningococcal carrier state).

PE

VS: normal. PE: muscular male in no acute distress; no jaundice, hepatomegaly, spider angiomas, or parotid enlargement; nonpruritic maculopapular **rash** on chest and **petechial hemorrhages** on limbs.

Labs

AST and ALT moderately **increased**. UA: **proteinuria**. CBC: **thrombocytopenia**.

Imaging

CXR/KUB: normal.

Treatment

Switch to ceftriaxone or ciprofloxacin for eradication of meningococcal carrier state.

Discussion

Rifampin is an antituberculous drug that acts by inhibiting DNA-dependent RNA polymerase. One of its major drawbacks is the rapid development of resistance if used alone. Other side effects include **discoloration of urine and sweat** with a yellowish-orange hue, **hepatic damage, skin rash, thrombocytopenia, tubulointerstitial nephritis**, and increased metabolism of anticoagulants and HIV protease inhibitors.

INFECTIOUS DISEASE

TOP SECRET

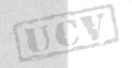

CASE 54

ID/CC

A 9-year-old girl is seen in the ER for vomiting.

HPI

Two days prior to admission she developed fever, chills, headache, myalgias, generalized fatigue, and cough. She was taken by her parents to a pediatrician yesterday and given **oseltamivir (Tamiflu)** liquid suspension for the treatment of flu. After taking the first dose, she began to experience nausea that progressed to **vomiting**.

PE

VS: **fever** (39.0°C); **tachycardia** (HR 110). PE: normal.

Labs

CBC: leukocytosis.

Treatment

Symptomatic and supportive treatment; continue to administer Tamiflu and monitor for improvement in flu symptoms; discontinue use if vomiting persists despite use of antiemetics.

Discussion

Oseltamivir is used for the treatment of **influenza types A and B** in adults and children; it decreases the duration and severity of flu symptoms if taken within 24 to 48 hours after symptoms begin. Along with **zanamivir**, it comprises a class of antiviral drugs called **neuroaminidase inhibitors**, which block the release of progeny viruses from infected cells. The most common adverse effect of oseltamivir is **vomiting**, which generally occurs only once and improves with continued dosing. Other events reported include **abdominal pain, epistaxis**, and **conjunctivitis**. Zanamivir can worsen pulmonary symptoms by decreasing peak expiratory flow rates in patients with underlying asthma or COPD.

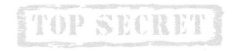

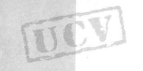

CASE 55

ID/CC

A 19-year-old **red-haired** female visits her dermatologist at a local clinic because of a **rash** that appeared after she spent the **sunny** weekend hiking without sun block protection.

HPI

Two months ago, her dermatologist put her on low-dose **tetracycline** to prevent acne flare-ups.

PE

VS: normal. PE: patient **blue-eyed** and **fair-skinned**; red, nonpruritic, **maculopapular rash** that blanches on pressure on "V" of the anterior neck, posterior neck, forearms, hands, and face, sparing rest of body (rash is on sun-exposed areas of body); chest, abdomen, and neurologic exams fail to disclose pathology.

Labs

CBC/Lytes: normal. LFTs within normal limits. UA: mild **proteinuria**.

Treatment

Sun protection, both mechanical and pharmacologic, while taking tetracycline.

Discussion

Tetracyclines are bacteriostatic antibiotics that bind to the 30S ribosomal unit, blocking synthesis of protein by preventing attachment of aminoacyl-tRNA. If they are taken with alkaline foods such as milk and antacids, GI absorption is decreased. Tetracycline is used both therapeutically and prophylactically for chlamydial genitourinary infections, Lyme disease, tularemia, cholera, and acne. Other side effects include **brownish discoloration of the teeth in children** (contraindicated in pregnancy), **photosensitivity**, aminoaciduria, proteinuria, phosphaturia, acidosis, and glycosuria (a Fanconi-like syndrome associated with "expired" tetracycline).

INFECTIOUS DISEASE

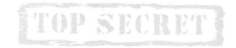

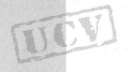

ID/CC   An asymptomatic **HIV-positive** 29-year-old male visits his infectious-disease specialist for a routine checkup; after determining his **CD4 count** **(410)**, the physician decides to start him on oral **zidovudine** (AZT) at a dosage of 600 mg/day.

HPI   Two months later, he returns to the doctor's office feeling very **tired** (due to anemia); he has also had two URIs and yesterday started **bleeding from his gums** (due to thrombocytopenia).

PE   VS: slight tachycardia. PE: marked **pallor**; **disseminated petechiae** on arms and legs.

Labs   CBC: **decreased platelets** (THROMBOCYTOPENIA); **decreased WBCs** (NEUTROPENIA); **decreased RBCs** (ANEMIA).

Treatment   Consider adding erythropoieitin or switch to an alternative antiviral such as zalcitabine.

Discussion   AZT is a nucleoside analog antiretroviral agent that acts by inhibiting viral DNA chain elongation. It is used alone or in combination with other nucleoside analogs for the treatment of symptomatic or asymptomatic HIV infections. To prevent resistance, a protease inhibitor is also added to the regimen. Common side effects include anorexia, nausea, vomiting, fatigue, and insomnia. Nail hyperpigmentation, myopathy, lactic acidosis, and hepatic toxicity may also result from chronic AZT therapy.

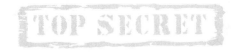

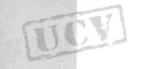

CASE 57

ID/CC

A 59-year-old female visits her family doctor complaining of **chronic fatigue**, **muscle weakness**, and **cramps**.

HPI

She has been receiving **furosemide** for the treatment of essential hypertension for more than 1 year.

PE

VS: **tachycardia**. PE: **dehydration**; somnolence; muscle weakness; deep tendon reflexes slow.

Labs

Elevated uric acid. Lytes: **decreased potassium and magnesium**. ECG: flattened T waves and prominent U waves (due to hypokalemia).

Treatment

Treatment consists of replacement of fluid and electrolyte losses. Monitor ECG for cardiac abnormalities.

Discussion

Significant dehydration and electrolyte imbalance may occur in loop diuretic overdose. These compounds (**furosemide, bumetanide, and ethacrynic acid**) are potent diuretics that inhibit the Na/K/2Cl transport system, which can result in **hypokalemic metabolic alkalosis**. Potassium replacement and correction of hypovolemia can reverse this toxicity. Additional **adverse effects** include **ototoxicity, hyperuricemia, allergic reactions** (except for ethacrynic acid which is not sulfa-derived) and **hypomagnesemia**.

NEPHROLOGY/UROLOGY

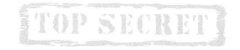

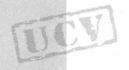

CASE 58

ID/CC
A 40-year-old woman who suffers from **chronic arthritis and headache** for which she takes several types of painkillers containing **phenacetin** says she had an episode of severe, colicky pain in the right lumbar region in the morning.

HPI
She adds that the pain radiated to the groin, her **urine was bloody**, and she **passed a small piece of soft tissue**, after which the pain subsided. The patient has not consumed any fluids since this episode. She also has a history of **recurrent UTIs**.

PE
VS: no fever; hypertension. PE: **anemia**; neither kidney palpable.

Labs
CBC: normocytic, normochromic anemia. **Serum creatinine and BUN elevated**. UA: **gross hematuria**; sediment with no crystals. Tissue that patient passed measures about 4 mm and is **gray and necrotic**; no crystalline material demonstrated.

Imaging
IVP: classic "ring sign" of papillary necrosis—**radiolucent, sloughed papilla surrounded by radiodense contrast material in calyx**. US abdomen: bilaterally small kidneys. CT: presence of papillary necrosis.

Micro Pathology
Papillary necrosis and tubulointerstitial inflammation on renal biopsy.

Treatment
Total **cessation of analgesic use**, adequate hydration, and control of hypertension. Regular surveillance of urine cytology will detect uroepithelial tumors, which may arise after discontinuation of analgesic agent.

Discussion
Renal papillary necrosis is seen in **middle-age females** with **migraines or rheumatic diseases** who take **large amounts of analgesics**. Usually there is a **psychological component** in the compulsion to take them.

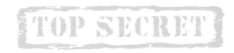

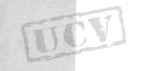

CASE 59

ID/CC

A 76-year-old female comes to her family doctor complaining of **constipation** and epigastric pain as well as **weakness** and painful **muscle cramps** (due to hypokalemia).

HPI

She has a history of hypertension, for which she has been taking propranolol and **hydrochlorothiazide** for the past several months.

PE

VS: mild hypertension (BP 145/90); no fever. PE: well hydrated; funduscopic exam shows hypertensive retinopathy grade II; no increase in JVP; no masses in neck; no carotid bruit; soft S3 heard; no hepatomegaly; no pitting edema of lower legs; **deep tendon reflexes hypoactive** (due to hypokalemia).

Labs

Hyperglycemia; increased BUN. Lytes: **hypokalemia; hyponatremia. Hyperlipidemia; hyperuricemia; hypomagnesemia; hypercalcemia.** UA: proteinuria; high specific gravity. ABGs: **metabolic alkalosis.** ECG: S-T segment depression; broad, flat T waves; U waves (due to hypokalemia).

Treatment

Potassium-rich foods (chickpeas, bananas, papaya, citrus fruits, prunes), potassium supplement, or switch to potassium-sparing diuretics such as spironolactone and triamterene.

Discussion

Thiazides, the most commonly used diuretics (of which hydrochlorothiazide is the prototype), are sulfonamide derivatives that act by **inhibiting sodium chloride reabsorption primarily in the early distal tubule.** They are used mainly in congestive heart failure, edematous states, and hypertension (they have a mild vasodilating effect). The hyperuricemia induced by thiazide diuretics can also precipitate bouts of gout.

NEPHROLOGY/UROLOGY

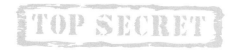

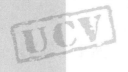

ID/CC
A 48-year-old patient being treated for a large abscess in his lower back develops **oliguria, hematuria**, and an extensive **erythematous skin rash**.

HPI
The patient has been treated according to culture and sensitivity of the pus from the abscess against *Staphylococcus aureus* with **methicillin**. He has no history of allergy to any medications.

PE
VS: fever (38.2°C); mild tachycardia. PE: erythematous **skin rash**; rales auscultated over left lung base.

Labs
Increased serum creatinine and **BUN**. CBC: eosinophilia. Blood culture sterile. UA: mild **proteinuria; sterile pyuria**; urinary sediment shows abundant eosinophils and no bacteria.

Imaging
US, abdomen: normal kidneys.

Micro Pathology
Renal biopsy shows evidence of **tubulointerstitial disease**; inflammatory infiltrate in interstitium consists of a large number of eosinophils in addition to neutrophils, lymphocytes, and plasma cells.

Treatment
Alternative antibiotic therapy and supportive management; cessation of offending drug often reverses disease.

Discussion
Drugs commonly associated with acute tubulointerstitial disease include penicillin, ampicillin, thiazides, rifampin, methicillin, and cimetidine. This type II hypersensitivity reaction is often reversed with cessation of offending drug; if it is not reversed, it may progress to renal failure.

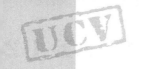

CASE 61

ID/CC   A 50-year-old male presents with **flushed skin, headaches, upset stomach, photophobia,** and **blue-tinted vision.**

HPI   He has been diagnosed with **erectile dysfunction** in the past and is currently on **sildenafil** (Viagra). He has no history of **diabetes** or of **cardiovascular, prostate,** or **anxiety problems.** He also takes cimetidine regularly for acid reflux.

PE   VS: **hypotension** (BP 90/50). PE: **plethoric** face; **nasal congestion.**

Labs   CBC/Lytes: normal. LFTs normal. ECG: normal.

Treatment   Adjust medications as necessary to prevent **cytochrome P450 interactions** with sildenafil. In this case, switch the patient from cimetidine to another H$_2$ receptor blocking agent with fewer interactions (such as ranitidine).

Discussion   Sildenafil, which acts by inhibiting phosphodiesterase, enhances the effect of **nitric oxide**, an endogenous **vasodilator** that relaxes penile smooth muscle and allows blood to flow in, producing an erection. Side effects are dose-related. Sildenafil is **absolutely contraindicated** when **nitrates** are used for treatment of angina and should be used cautiously in patients taking **antihypertensive medications** or with preexisting cardiovascular disease. Reported deaths due to sildenafil are typically **cardiovascular events in elderly men** (> 65 years of age). Sildenafil is metabolized by the liver via the **cytochrome P450 system** and should be used cautiously in patients taking cimetidine, erythromycin, rifampin, and ketoconazole.

NEPHROLOGY/UROLOGY

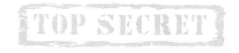

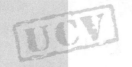

CASE 62

ID/CC A 28-year-old female is started on **amantadine prophylaxis**; she teaches at a school where there has been an **influenza** outbreak.

HPI One week later, she started feeling **dizzy** and having **problems walking normally** (ATAXIA). An ENT consult ruled out middle-ear causes of vertigo.

PE VS: **no fever**; remainder of vital signs normal. PE: **speech** somewhat **slurred; gait ataxic**; no focal neurologic signs.

Labs CBC/Lytes/UA: normal.

Imaging MR/CT: no intracranial pathology.

Treatment Discontinue amantadine. Amantadine is not effectively removed by dialysis because of its large volume of distribution.

Discussion Amantadine is an antiviral agent that blocks viral penetration and uncoating. It also causes the release of dopamine from intact nerve terminals (sometimes used for treatment of Parkinson's disease). It is used as **prophylaxis against influenza A**. Toxicity includes cerebellar problems such as **ataxic gait, slurred speech**, and **dizziness**. Elderly patients with renal insufficiency are more susceptible to toxicity.

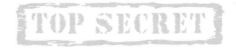

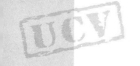

CASE 63

ID/CC

A 24-year-old female visits her physician because of **pain in her arm** after spending all day cleaning the basement of her house; x-rays taken as a routine procedure revealed a **linear fracture** of the right radius.

HPI

She is an epileptic who has been treated for 3 years with **phenytoin**. She states that she has been suffering from increasing **leg weakness** and persistent **lower back pain**.

PE

VS: normal. PE: **increase in size of gums** (GINGIVAL HYPERPLASIA); no neck masses; no lymphadenopathy; chest normal to auscultation; abdomen soft with no masses; no neurologic signs; **hirsutism** present; linear right radial fracture; **tenderness of lumbar vertebrae and pelvic rim**.

Labs

Megaloblastic anemia; BUN and creatinine normal; **glucose mildly elevated; increased alkaline phosphatase**; decreased levels of vitamin D; **hypocalcemia; hypophosphatemia**.

Imaging

XR: right radial fracture; **shortening of lumbar vertebrae; generalized osteopenia and Looser's lines** (MILKMAN'S FRACTURES; PATHOGNOMONIC). DEXA: confirms presence of severe osteopenia.

Treatment

Switch to other antiepileptics; vitamin D and calcium and folate supplements; bisphosphonate therapy; treat fracture, physiotherapy.

Discussion

Phenytoin and, to a lesser extent, other antiepileptic drugs such as phenobarbital and carbamazepine may cause **vitamin D deficiency** with consequent development of osteomalacia (in adults) and rickets (in children). Fractures with minor trauma may be a presenting sign, as may bone pain and proximal muscle weakness.

NEUROLOGY

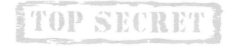

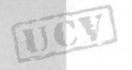

ID/CC   A 45-year-old **female** comes to her family physician for an evaluation of frequent URIs (due to neutropenia) and gum bleeding (due to thrombo cytopenia). She also complains of **double vision** (DIPLOPIA), nausea sleepiness, and **dry mouth** as well as difficulty walking.

HPI   She has been suffering from recurrent, severe, sharp pain on the left side of her face that radiates to the corner of her eye and is triggered by mas tication or cold exposure (TRIGEMINAL NEURALGIA). She has been taking **car bamazepine** for several months, during which time her attacks have been much less frequent.

PE   VS: normal. PE: well hydrated, oriented, and in no acute distress; **ataxic gait**; funduscopic exam normal except for mild **mydriasis**.

Labs   CBC: **decreased platelets; decreased neutrophil count**. Coagulation and bleeding time increased. LP: CSF normal. No evidence of multiple sclerosis on evoked-potential testing; **AST and ALT** moderately **increased**; serum carbamazepine level supratherapeutic (> 12 mg/dL).

Imaging   CT, brain: normal.

Treatment   Consider alternative treatment options for trigeminal neuralgia, such as baclofen, clonazepam, phenytoin, or valproic acid.

Discussion   Trigeminal neuralgia is sometimes seen in association with multiple scle rosis, primarily in younger patients. Carbamazepine is chemically similar to imipramine and has been used for trigeminal neuralgia as well as for the treatment of partial and tonic-clonic seizures.

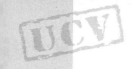

CASE 65

ID/CC A neonatologist is called upon to evaluate a newborn with multiple birth defects.

HPI The mother is a 17-year-old runaway who is homeless, had no prenatal care, and continued her habit of **getting drunk** two to three times a week **throughout her pregnancy**.

PE Low birth weight; small head size (MICROCEPHALY); facial flattening with epicanthal folds; small eyes (MICROPHTHALMOS); cardiac murmur (diagnosed as an atrial septal defect); positive Ortolani's sign on left hip and lack of complete hip abduction on that side; chest deformed (pectus excavatum).

Labs CBC: mild anemia. Increased AST and ALT.

Imaging CXR: cardiomegaly; pectus excavatum deformity. XR, hip: congenital dislocation of left hip.

Treatment No specific treatment available; treat each malformation/disease accordingly.

Discussion Alcohol is the leading cause of fetal malformations in the United States. Fetal alcohol syndrome may cause myriad abnormalities, both skeletal and visceral, but usually involves a triad of features: (1) craniofacial dysmorphology, including mild to moderate **microcephaly** and **maxillary hypoplasia**; (2) prenatal and postnatal **growth retardation**; and (3) CNS abnormalities, including **mental retardation**, with IQs often in the range of 50 to 70. In addition, fetal alcohol exposure leads to an increased incidence of **cardiac malformations**, including **patent ductus arteriosus** and **septal defects**. Risk is dose related.

NEUROLOGY

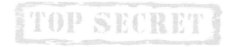

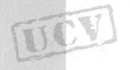

CASE 66

ID/CC A 23-year-old female is terrified after reportedly seeing grotesque monsters trying to kill her while she had her left dislocated shoulder reduced.

HPI She injured her shoulder while rock climbing in Colorado. The doctor was called upon to see her immediately after the accident. She did not suffer major injuries but had a dislocated shoulder and was not cooperative enough to tolerate the procedure (reduction) without medication, so he anesthetized her with **ketamine**, atropine, and diazepam.

Imaging X-rays at time of injury showed an anterior shoulder dislocation.

Treatment Benzodiazepines (e.g., diazepam) reduce the adverse effects of ketamine.

Discussion Ketamine is an arylcyclohexylamine that produces a **dissociative anesthesia**; the patient has open eyes, and muscle tone is preserved (with sufficient analgesia to do major surgery and total amnesia). Its major side effect is **vivid hallucinations**, sometimes terrifying, upon arousal, mostly in adults. It is widely used in developing countries, in rural areas where there is no available anesthesiologist, and in short pediatric procedures (abscess debridement, burn wounds, dressing changes, etc.) because of its relative safety and lack of life-threatening side effects (such as respiratory depression, which is common with other anesthetics). However, it also causes cardiac stimulation with increased blood pressure and tachycardia.

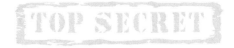

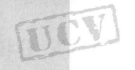
ɔ/CC

An 82-year-old male complains to his doctor about chronic **nausea** and vomiting, **loss of appetite**, and **altered taste perception** as well as **involuntary tremors, chewing, and grimacing movements** (DYSKINESIA).

IPI

The patient also states he has been having **palpitations** and **insomnia**. He suffers from Parkinson's disease and has been taking **levodopa** for a long time.

E

VS: **tachycardia** (HR 115); **postural hypotension**. PE: patient thin; typical parkinsonian gait; masklike facies; pill-rolling tremor of hands; **choreiform movements** of head and hands; grimacing facial movements.

abs

CBC/PBS: **Coombs' test positive**; no hemolytic anemia. ECG: **premature ventricular contractions** (cause of palpitations). Urine and saliva are brownish in color.

ʀeatment

Minimize side effects by taking drug with meals or in smaller doses. Often, administration of carbidopa diminishes side effects. Tolerance to emetic effect may also develop. Antiemetics may be given, but these may reduce antiparkinsonian effects.

ⅰscussion

Dopamine cannot cross the blood-brain barrier; however, levodopa, a precursor of dopamine, does. When this drug is administered, it is usually given in combination with carbidopa, an inhibitor of the peripheral dopa decarboxylase (thus increasing the half-life and plasma levels of levodopa). Dyskinesias are a common side effect, as are GI symptoms (nausea and vomiting) and postural hypotension. Arrhythmias, anxiety, depression, insomnia, and confusion have also been reported. The dose of levodopa must be slowly decreased, since **abrupt cessation** may result in an **akinetic state**. Many patients eventually experience a decline in efficacy with levodopa/carbidopa. They may develop an "on-off" phenomenon in which they suddenly lose activity of the levodopa and are "frozen." Other patients experience a more gradual decline in which the levodopa effect lasts for shorter periods of time.

NEUROLOGY

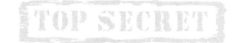

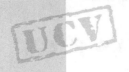

CASE 68

ID/CC

A 16-year-old female patient undergoes **surgery** to remove an inflamed appendix and has a rare anesthesia complication.

HPI

The father states that the patient's paternal uncle died of an anesthetic complication. The patient has had no prior surgery and received general anesthesia in the form of **halothane** and **succinylcholine**.

PE

VS: very high **fever** (39.8°C); **hypertension** (BP 150/95). PE: generalized **muscular rigidity** with difficulty breathing, anxiety, and marked sweating.

Labs

CBC: leukocytosis with neutrophilia. Lytes: **hyperkalemia**. ABGs: metabolic acidosis. Elevated CK.

Treatment

Immediate treatment to lower body temperature, control acidosis, and restore electrolyte balance is critical to survival. **IV dantrolene** relaxes skeletal muscle by inhibiting release of calcium from sarcoplasmic reticulum. This allows muscle to relax and limits hyperthermia from muscle hyperactivity.

Discussion

Malignant hyperthermia is a highly lethal, genetically determined **myopathy** (**autosomal-dominant** trait). It is triggered by inhalation anesthetics (more commonly halothane), particularly those coupled with succinylcholine. The syndrome includes **tachycardia**, **hypertension**, **acidosis**, **hyperkalemia**, and **muscle rigidity**, and it appears to be related to excess myoplasmic calcium.

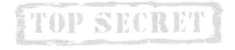

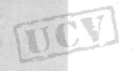

CASE 69

/CC

A 32-year-old male is brought by his wife to the family care center of the community because of increasing **tremors, slowing of movements** (BRADYKINESIA), and **postural instability**.

PI

The patient works as a **chemist** at a leading pharmaceutical research company in Northern California and has a long-standing history of **drug abuse requiring hospitalization**.

E

VS: normal. PE: flat facies; **resting tremor; cogwheel rigidity**; impaired capacity for voluntary motor activity; speech slow, as are voluntary movements.

naging

CT, head: no apparent intracranial pathology.

reatment

No effective therapy currently exists for treatment of drug-induced Parkinson's syndrome aside from discontinuation of offending drug.

iscussion

Several drugs may produce Parkinson-like symptoms, including haloperidol and phenothiazines, which block dopamine receptors, as well as reserpine and tetrabenazine, which deplete biogenic monoamines from their storage sites. In their attempts to produce "designer drugs" related to meperidine, "underground" chemists have also synthesized a compound, 1-methyl-4-phenyl-tetrahydrobiopteridine (MPTP). The toxicity of MPTP is produced by its oxidation to **MPP+** (a toxic compound), which selectively **destroys the dopaminergic neurons in the substantia nigra**.

NEUROLOGY

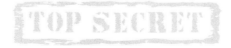

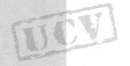

CASE 70

ID/CC	A 21-year-old male who emigrated to the United States 3 months ago visit a neighborhood medical clinic complaining of apprehension, tremors dizziness, **inability to walk properly, and double vision** (DIPLOPIA).
HPI	He is a newly diagnosed epileptic whose understanding of English is ver poor, so when his doctor prescribed one tablet of **phenytoin** ever 24 hours, he thought the doctor meant one tablet every 2 to 4 hours.
PE	VS: hypotension; bradycardia. PE: bilateral nystagmus with sluggis pupils; patient is slightly lethargic; ataxic gait; dysarthria.
Labs	CBC: megaloblastic anemia. Moderate increases in AST and ALT. ECG sinus bradycardia. Serum phenytoin level supratherapeutic.
Imaging	CXR: normal. CT, head: no intracranial pathology seen.
Treatment	Gastric lavage or activated charcoal if acute overdose. Stop treatmen temporarily; then resume at proper dosage.
Discussion	Overdose may be lethal owing to the ability of phenytoin to induc CNS, cardiac, and respiratory depression. Certain drugs, such as INH cimetidine, and sulfonamides, can increase phenytoin levels by inhibit ing the microsome enzymes that are responsible for the metabolism c phenytoin. The rate of hydroxylation of phenytoin also varies amon individuals as a result of genetic differences.

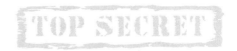

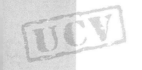
ID/CC

A 65-year-old female with long-standing **osteoarthritis** presents with **bilateral lower extremity swelling**.

HPI

For the last 2 months, she has been taking **celecoxib** for relief of joint pain and inflammation.

PE

VS: normal. PE: JVP normal; S1 and S2 auscultated normally without any murmurs, gallops, or rubs; **mild, bilateral pitting lower extremity edema**.

Labs

CBC/Lytes: normal. LFTs normal. ECG: normal.

Treatment

Monitor for worsening edema; provide temporary relief with diuretics; may need to switch to an alternative NSAID.

Discussion

Celecoxib is a nonsteroidal anti-inflammatory drug (NSAID) used to treat **osteoarthritis** and adult **rheumatoid arthritis**. Recently, it has also been used to reduce the number of **colorectal polyps** in patients with **familial adenomatous polyposis (FAP)** and shows promise in treating GI cancers. Celecoxib works by inhibiting **cyclooxygenase-2 (COX-2)**, but unlike other NSAIDs, it does not inhibit COX-1. As a result, there is a postulated **reduction in the incidence of upper GI ulcers** as compared to aspirin, ibuprofen, and naproxen, as well as less interference with blood platelets/clotting. Celecoxib is contraindicated in patients who are allergic to sulfa drugs or aspirin. It can also cause **liver damage** and/or **edema**. The efficacy of **thiazide diuretics, loop diuretics, and ACE inhibitors** is **diminished** by celecoxib.

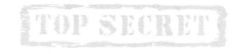

ORTHOPEDICS

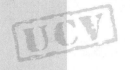

ID/CC An 18-year-old high-school dropout is brought to the ER because of marked **restlessness, euphoria, anxiety, tachycardia, paranoia,** and **agitation.**

HPI The patient is a known **drug abuser** with an otherwise unremarkable medical history.

PE VS: marked **hypertension** (BP 185/100); **tachycardia** (HR 165). PE **diaphoresis; tremor.**

Labs Amphetamine levels are detectable in **urine** and gastric samples. UA **occult hemoglobin** (due to **rhabdomyolysis** with **myoglobinuria**).

Treatment Treat agitation, seizures, and coma if they occur; treat hypertension with benzodiazepines; if refractory or severe, use IV vasodilator such as phentolamine or nitroprusside. Propranolol is used to prevent tachyarrhythmias.

Discussion A variety of amphetamines are used clinically, including methylphenidate (Ritalin) for attention deficit hyperactivity disorder (ADHD). However many of these drugs are commonly abused as well. Such agents activate CNS via peripheral release of catecholamines, inhibition of reuptake mechanisms, or inhibition of monoamine oxidase enzymes. Excretion is dependent on urine pH, with optimal excretion occurring in acidified urine.

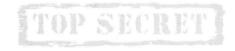

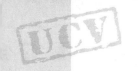

PSYCHOPHARMACOLOGY

ID/CC A 20-year-old medical student is brought to the emergency room because his roommate noticed that he had been **sleeping all day** and awakening from time to time with **nightmares**; the patient then stated that **he wanted to shoot himself** and began to look for a gun.

HPI He had just finished end-of-year exams in all his subjects, for which he had studied late into the night and had taken **methylphenidate** daily for several weeks.

PE VS: mild tachycardia. PE: well-oriented with respect to time, person, and place but very **lethargic** and complains of a severe **headache**; funduscopic exam normal; no increased JVP; no neck masses; lungs clear; heart sounds with no murmurs; abdomen soft and nontender with no masses; peristaltic sounds increased (patient complains of abdominal cramps when these are heard).

Labs Routine lab exams fail to disclose abnormality; urine tox screen shows only trace amounts of amphetamine.

Imaging CXR: no cardiopulmonary pathology apparent.

Treatment Hospitalization due to risk of suicide, antidepressants, supportive treatment.

Discussion Amphetamines are used recreationally for their ability to produce a sense of well-being and euphoria, with sympathetic stimulation. There are also some medical indications for their use, such as hyperactive child syndrome. Amphetamines may be abused orally or parenterally or may be smoked. **Withdrawal symptoms** include lethargy, **suicidal thoughts, profound depression**, intestinal colic, headache, sleepiness, and nightmares.

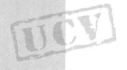

CASE 74

ID/CC A 19-year-old **epileptic** student is brought by ambulance to the emergency room in a **coma** after being found on the floor of her apartment.

HPI She had been feeling depressed for several months and, according to her roommate, had just broken up with her boyfriend. She took a **whole bottle of her antiepileptic pills** at once (**phenobarbital**).

PE She was brought to the ER **unconscious, hypotensive, hypothermic** (35°C), and **bradypneic**. PE: no response to verbal stimulation; reacts only to painful stimuli; **bullae** on lower legs; deep tendon **reflexes slow** (HYPOREFLEXIA).

Labs ABGs: pronounced **hypoxemia** and **respiratory acidosis. Blood alcohol level also increased**. ECG: sinus bradycardia.

Imaging CXR: no evidence of aspiration (a common complication of sedative overdose due to diminished gag reflex and altered consciousness).

Gross Pathology Globus pallidus necrosis with pulmonary and cerebral edema.

Treatment Airway maintenance; oxygen; assisted ventilation; gastric lavage cathartics; alkalinization of urine; warming blankets; consider pressors hemodialysis or hemoperfusion. **Flumazenil reverses benzodiazepine overdose but not barbiturate overdose**.

Discussion Barbiturates facilitate GABA action by increasing the duration of the chloride channel opening; they are used as antianxiety drugs, in sleep disorders, and in anesthesia. Barbiturates **induce the cytochrome P450 system** of liver microsomal enzymes, thereby affecting the metabolism of several drugs. In overdose, death may ensue due to severe **respiratory depression** or **aspiration pneumonia**.

TOP SECRET

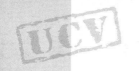

CASE 75

ID/CC

A 6-year-old-girl is brought to the pediatric emergency room because she accidentally consumed large quantities of her sister's **"Vivarin"** stimulant pills.

HPI

The child, a healthy girl with no previous medical history, mistook the pills for candy, as they were in a non-child proof container in the kitchen cabinet.

PE

VS: **tachycardia** (HR 175); **hypotension** (BP 115/60). PE: **extreme restlessness, tremors**, and **nausea**.

Labs

CBC/Lytes/UA: normal. SMA-7 normal.

Imaging

CXR/KUB: within normal limits for age.

Treatment

Monitor patient for ECG changes. Treat tachycardia and possible hypotension due to excess β_1 and β_2 stimulation with propranolol or esmolol.

Discussion

Caffeine is widely used as an appetite and **sleep suppressant** and as a **diuretic**. It has a wide therapeutic index; however, serious toxicity may result from accidental ingestion of large quantities. Beta-blockers effectively reverse the cardiotoxic effects of excess catecholamine release and stimulation.

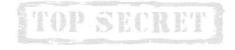

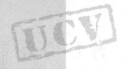
ID/CC   A 14-year old boy is brought to the ER by his anxious mother for mild somnolence, mild stupor, and mild motor dysfunction. The patient initially answers negatively to questions about drug use.

HPI   Upon further private questioning, he reveals that he had been "smoking a joint."

PE   VS: tachycardia; mild tachypnea. PE: conjunctiva red and injected.

Labs   UA: presence of cannabinoids.

Treatment   No specific therapy; reassurance; benzodiazepines as needed for anxiety.

Discussion   The primary psychoactive agent in marijuana is delta-9-tetrahydro cannabinol, which is released during pyrolysis (smoking) of *Cannabis sativa*. Acute cannabis intoxication usually consists of a subjective perception of relaxation and mild euphoria accompanied by mild impairment in thinking, concentration, and perceptual and psycho social functions. Chronic abusers may lose interest in common socially desirable goals. Therapeutic effects include treatment for glaucoma, prevention of emesis associated with cancer chemotherapy, and appetite stimulation ("THE MUNCHIES").

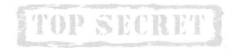

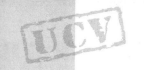

CASE 77

ID/CC

A 24-year-old female of Ashkenazi Jewish background complains to her family doctor of **repeated URIs** (due to neutropenia), increasing **fatigue, muscle aches, and headaches.**

HPI

She had been showing flattening of affect, suspiciousness, a delusional mood, and auditory hallucinations that were diagnosed as **schizophrenia** 3 years ago. She was recently switched to clozapine because other antipsychotics were unsuccessful.

PE

VS: **fever**; tachycardia (HR 165). PE: patient in obvious discomfort; **pallor** (due to anemia); conscious and oriented to person, place, and time; **petechiae** (due to thrombocytopenia) on chest and arms; cardiopulmonary, abdominal, and genital exams normal; no extrapyramidal signs.

Labs

CBC: agranulocytosis.

Imaging

CXR: No signs of lung infection.

Treatment

Discontinue clozapine and institute alternate pharmacotherapy; granulocyte colony-stimulating factor in severe cases.

Discussion

Clozapine is used for the treatment of schizophrenia and psychotic disorders that are unresponsive to other therapy. It blocks D_1, D_2, and D_4 dopamine receptors as well as serotonin receptors. Because of its low affinity for D_2 receptors, clozapine causes few extrapyramidal symptoms. Agranulocytosis occurs in < 2% of patients, but all patients must receive weekly blood counts to monitor for this potentially lethal effect. Other side effects include seizures, sedation, and anticholinergic symptoms. Agranulocytosis usually reverses with discontinuation of clozapine.

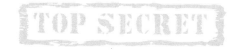

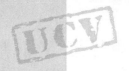

CASE 78

ID/CC   A 32-year-old stockbroker is brought to the ER after police find him **hiding in an alley**.

HPI   The patient had been at a **party** with several friends. He admits to indulging in cocaine from a new dealer for the past 6 hours.

PE   VS: **hypertension** (BP 180/95); **tachycardia** (HR 160). PE: **restless, mal nourished**, and **disoriented**.

Treatment   Monitor vital signs and ECG for several hours. There are no specific antidotes for cocaine use. Control hypertension with benzodiazepine and **phentolamines**; avoid beta-blockers to prevent paradoxical hyper tension (from unopposed alpha-vasoconstriction). In severe cases, trea dysrhythmias with IV sodium bicarbonate or lidocaine. Dialysis and hemoperfusion are not effective.

Discussion   Cocaine is a CNS stimulant and an inhibitor of neuronal catecholamine reuptake mechanisms; hence, its use results in a state of generalized sympathetic stimulation, with typical symptoms including **euphoria anxiety, psychosis**, and **hyperactivity**. Severe **hypertension, ventricu lar tachycardia**, or **fibrillation** may also occur. **Angina pectoris** in a young, healthy person is suggestive of cocaine use. **Myocardial infarc tion** secondary to **coronary vasospasm** and thrombosis have been described as well.

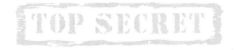

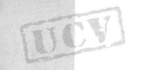

CASE 79

ID/CC   A 36-year-old male, an ENT doctor, tells his psychiatrist that he has been feeling terribly **depressed** and **anxious** over the last 3 weeks.

HPI   The patient has been in good health, but he recently entered into a **drug rehabilitation program** to **wean** himself **off cocaine**.

PE   VS: tachycardia; BP normal; no fever. PE: patient expresses concern over his increasing **lethargy, depression, hunger,** and **extreme cravings for stimulants** such as cocaine.

Labs   Basic lab work and tox screen are all within normal limits. ECG: sinus tachycardia.

Treatment   No definitive treatment exists to alleviate symptoms of cocaine withdrawal and associated cravings. Bromocriptine, a dopamine agonist that is used in Parkinson's disease, has been reported to diminish cocaine cravings.

Discussion   Symptoms of cocaine withdrawal may be due to enhanced sensitivity of inhibitory receptors on dopaminergic neurons. In contrast to mild physiologic withdrawal signs and symptoms, cocaine produces marked psychological dependency and behavioral withdrawal symptoms.

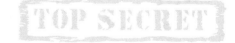

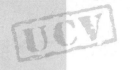

CASE 80

ID/CC
A 35-year-old plastic **surgeon** is rushed to the hospital by his wife after he is found lying comatose in his bed with a couple of **syringes lying on the floor** and his sleeve rolled up.

HPI
His wife states that her husband had been having serious financial problems; she has suspected drug use in light of recent **personality and mood changes**.

PE
On admission to ER, patient had a tonic-clonic **seizure; respiratory depression**; bradycardia; stupor; **pupils very constricted** (PINPOINT PUPILS); cold skin; hypotension; marked hyporeflexia; hypoactive bowel sounds; **needle "train track" marks** (stigmata of multiple previous injections).

Labs
ABGs: hypoxemia; hypercapnia; respiratory acidosis. Urine tox screen positive for opioids.

Imaging
CXR: **noncardiogenic pulmonary edema** (edema without cardiomegaly).

Gross Pathology
Pulmonary congestion and edema; inflammatory neutrophilic infiltrate of arteries in brain and lung.

Micro Pathology
Brain cell swelling due to hypoxia.

Treatment
Establish a patent airway, assist ventilation, correct acid-base disorders, hypothermia, and hypotension. **Naloxone** as specific antagonist (naloxone may induce rapid opiate withdrawal), with follow-up in ICU.

Discussion
Heroin is a synthetic derivative of morphine that is abused as a recreational drug. Health professionals have a higher incidence of opioid abuse, generally abusing medical opioids. Heroin abuse is a complex social disease that is linked with violence, prostitution, crime, antisocial behavior, and premature death; it may result in fatal overdose, endocarditis, fungal infections, abscess formation, anaphylaxis, and HIV transmission. Death may result from aspiration of gastric contents or from apnea.

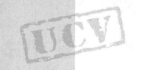
CASE 81

ID/CC

A 26-year-old female who models for photography magazines is referred to the dermatologist by her family doctor because of **persistent acne** that has been unresponsive to the usual treatment.

HPI

She also complains of **constant thirst**, dryness of the mouth, and **frequent urination**. She has been diagnosed with **bipolar affective disorder** with **manic** predominance and was recently started on **lithium therapy**.

PE

Sensorium normal; oriented and cooperative; fine resting tremor of hands; **mouth is dry**; no signs of present depression or mania; face shows presence of **severe cystic acne** on chin, forehead, and upper chest with **folliculitis**; mucous membranes dry.

Labs

CBC: **leukocytosis**. Lytes: mild hyponatremia. BUN and creatinine normal; pregnancy test negative. ECG: T-wave inversion. Supratherapeutic lithium levels detected in blood.

Treatment

Decrease or discontinue lithium use; severe cases may need dialysis; treat acne with isotretinoin (teratogenic), tetracycline, or benzoyl peroxide.

Discussion

Lithium is the preferred treatment for the manic stage of bipolar affective disorder; however, its mechanism of action on mood stability is still unclear. One possibility revolves around lithium's effects on the IP_3 second-messenger system in the brain. The onset of action may take several days, and side effects may be very bothersome, such as persistent polyuria and polydipsia (ADH antagonism), weight gain, and severe acne. It is contraindicated in pregnancy due to its teratogenic effect.

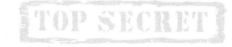

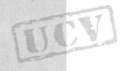

ID/CC   A 40-year-old male was brought into the ER by his sister, who reported that he had dropped by her apartment acting "drunk" and agitated.

HPI   The patient was diagnosed as suffering from major depressive disorder 1 month ago and had been on phenelzine (MAO inhibitor) for 3 weeks. He was switched to paroxetine (a selective serotonin reuptake inhibitor or SSRI) last week.

PE   VS: fever (39.0°C); hypertension (BP 150/100); tachycardia (HR 110) tachypnea (RR 30). PE: disoriented; agitated, diaphoretic; neurologic exam reveals hyperreflexia, resting hand tremor, and rigid extremities.

Labs   ABGs: metabolic acidosis.

Treatment External cooling; supportive care; IV benzodiazepines for agitation and seizures; antihypertensives.

Discussion Serotonin syndrome is characterized by an excess of serotonin in the bloodstream. The combination most frequently leading to serotonin syndrome is a monoamine oxidase (MAO) inhibitor given with an SSRI. Other drugs that can precipitate serotonin syndrome in combination with an MAO inhibitor or an SSRI include opioids (dextromethorphan, meperidine) and street drugs such as cocaine and LSD. In severe cases serotonin syndrome progresses to seizures, disseminated intravascular coagulation (DIC), renal failure, coma, and death. Tyramine-containing foods such as cheeses and beer in combination with an MAO inhibitor, can also cause a hypertensive crisis. Patients should stop using an MAO inhibitor at least 14 days before starting SSRI therapy.

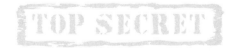

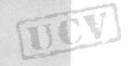
CASE 83

ID/CC

A 43-year-old art consultant in an advertising agency is brought to the emergency room with **severe headache, palpitations, ringing in her ears**, and **sweating**; she had been **drinking** and dining at a French restaurant.

HPI

Over the past several months she had seen several physicians for a variety of complaints before finally being diagnosed with **hypochondriasis** and given medication for it (**tranylcypromine**).

PE

VS: tachycardia; **hypertension** (BP 180/120); no fever. PE: **pupils dilated**; no papilledema; no signs of long-standing hypertensive retinopathy; no goiter (hyperthyroidism may lead to hypertensive crises).

Labs

CBC/Lytes: normal. LFTs normal; no vanillylmandelic acid in urine (seen in pheochromocytoma). UA: normal.

Imaging

CXR: normal.

Treatment

Gastric lavage; activated charcoal; treat hypertensive crisis with alpha-blockers to avoid producing hypotension; external cooling to manage hyperthermia. Avoid tyramine-containing foods.

Discussion

Monoamine oxidase (MAO) is an enzyme that degrades catecholamines. When inhibited, catecholamine and serotonin levels increase. MAO inhibitors such as **tranylcypromine**, and **phenelzine** are used to treat **anxiety, hypochondriasis**, and **atypical depressions. Tyramine** is a catecholamine food precursor (normally degraded by monoamine oxidase) found in **fermented meats, cheeses, beer, and red wine**. When taken together, tyramine and MAO inhibitors rapidly elevate blood pressure with possible encephalopathy and stroke.

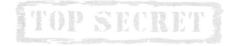

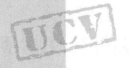

CASE 84

ID/CC   A 27-year-old female is brought to the emergency room by her mother because of a **high fever** and **muscle rigidity**.

HPI   The patient's mother reports that her daughter is being treated with **antipsychotics** for schizophrenia but is otherwise in good health.

PE   VS: **tachycardia** (HR 165); **hypotension** (BP 100/50); **fever**. PE: **confused** with an altered level of consciousness; pallor; **diaphoresis** (due to autonomic instability); marked rigidity of all muscle groups.

Labs   CBC: **leukocytosis**. Increased **CK** (indicates muscle damage). ABGs: metabolic **acidosis**.

Treatment   Treat muscle rigidity with **diazepam** and **initiate rapid cooling** to prevent brain damage (fever may reach dangerous levels). **Dantrolene, dopamine** agonists (bromocriptine) may be effective. Respiratory support.

Discussion   Neuroleptic malignant syndrome is a life-threatening complication characterized by generalized rigidity and high fever that occur in certain patients with an idiosyncratic reaction to antipsychotics, such as haloperidol and trifluoperazine hydrochloride. The onset of symptoms is usually within a couple of weeks after the drug is started; diminished iron reserves and dehydration are predisposing factors.

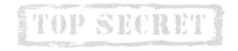

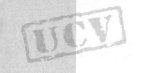

CASE 85

ID/CC

A 48-year-old male complains to his doctor about increasing anxiety, **insomnia, irritability,** and **severe cravings** for cigarettes and food.

HPI

The patient, a two-pack-a-day smoker for 20 years, recently **quit smoking.** He claims that he is **no longer able to relax** and has been having problems with his wife and at work due to impulsiveness.

PE

VS: **tachycardia** (HR 155); **hypertension** (BP 165/110). PE: patient **anxious** and **sweating.**

Labs

CBC: increased hematocrit. Hypertriglyceridemia; hypercholesterolemia.

Imaging

CXR: signs of chronic bronchitis and emphysema.

Treatment

Nicotine patches, nasal spray, or **gum** may be helpful in weaning smokers from nicotine addiction. **Bupropion** has been shown to be effective.

Discussion

Nicotine produces **serious addiction** and long-lasting cravings upon quitting. Nicotine produces euphoriant effects; however, tolerance develops rapidly. The psychological dependence of nicotine is very severe and a major impediment to quitting the tobacco habit. It is sometimes stronger than the physiologic dependence.

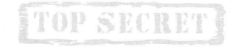

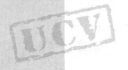

CASE 86

ID/CC
A 32-year-old male, the lead drummer of a popular rock band, presents to the emergency room with **high fever, a running nose**, and **severe diarrhea** as well as abdominal pain.

HPI
He is a chronic user of multiple drugs and had been a **heroin addict** for 2 years until two days ago, when he decided to quit.

PE
VS: **tachycardia** (HR 165); **hypertension** (BP 160/90). PE: patient has **lacrimation and rhinorrhea** and is thin, **anxious**, malnourished, and **sweating** profusely; generalized **piloerection** ("GOOSEBUMPS"); abdomen shows tenderness to deep palpation, but no muscle rigidity or peritoneal signs.

Labs
CBC/Lytes: normal.

Treatment
Treat volume deficit and electrolyte abnormalities resulting from diarrhea; **methadone** for symptomatic relief; **clonidine** to treat sympathetic hyperactivity; **benzodiazepines** for anxiety.

Discussion
Tolerance to opioids is a true cellular adaptive response on many levels including Ca^{2+} flux, G-protein synthesis, and adenyl cyclase inhibition. Withdrawal effects consist of **rhinorrhea, yawning, piloerection, lacrimation, diarrhea, vomiting, anxiety,** and **hostility**. These effects begin within 6 hours of the last dose and may last 4 to 5 days. Cravings for opiates may last for many years.

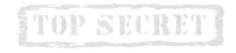

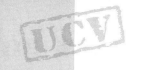

ID/CC

A 52-year-old college professor with a history of **schizophrenia** presents with **tremor and rigidity**.

HPI

The patient is **diabetic** and a **smoker** and has been receiving **antipsychotic** therapy for **many years**.

PE

Abnormal facial gestures, including **lip smacking, jaw muscle spasms**, and jerky movements around mouth; increased blinking frequency and difficulty with speech.

Labs

All labs normal.

Imaging

XR, skull: calcification of pineal gland.

Treatment

Decreasing dose or switching to atypical neuroleptics is first step. Benzodiazepine treatment can often improve GABAergic activity and therefore alleviate symptoms. Propranolol and calcium channel blockers may be of use.

Discussion

Tardive dyskinesia is a syndrome characterized by late-occurring abnormal **choreoathetoid movements**. It is often associated with antipsychotic drugs (e.g., dopamine blockers) and is estimated to affect about 30% of patients receiving treatment (males and females affected equally). Predisposing factors include older age, smoking, and diabetes. Advanced cases of tardive dyskinesia may be irreversible, so **early recognition of symptoms is critical**.

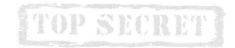

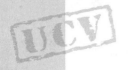

CASE 88

ID/CC A 26-year-old female is brought to the ER by her boss after **fainting** at work. The day before she had complained of a **dry mouth** along with **constipation and urinary retention**.

HPI She had a major manic episode of hyperactivity and productivity at work 2 months ago as well as auditory hallucinations, for which she was diagnosed with a schizoaffective disorder and has been undergoing treatment with the antipsychotic drug **thioridazine**.

PE VS: orthostatic hypotension; tachycardia (HR 108). PE: acute **depression**; **dryness of mouth**; inability to accommodate normally (with resultant blurred vision); funduscopic exam shows **pigmentary retinopathy** and **dilated pupils**; abdomen slightly distended with diminished peristaltic movements.

Labs Increased prolactin levels; hyperglycemia. ECG: flattened T wave; appearance of U waves; Q-T segment prolongation.

Treatment Discontinue offending drug.

Discussion Antipsychotic drugs such as thioridazine and chlorpromazine manifest a number of adverse effects, making drug compliance difficult. Muscarinic blockade produces typical anticholinergic effects such as tachycardia, loss of accommodation, urinary retention, and constipation. Alpha blockade produces **orthostatic hypotension**. Other side effects include **extrapyramidal signs** (AKATHISIA, TARDIVE DYSKINESIA, AKINESIA, DYSTONIA, CONVULSIONS). Pigmentary retinopathy is restricted to thioridazine use.

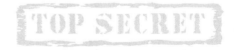

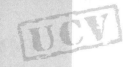

ID/CC

A 5-year-old male is rushed to the emergency department after his mother found him playing with her purse, where she carries her **antidepressants** (imipramine); she noticed that the boy had swallowed a handful of pills.

HPI

The child complained of **dry mouth, blurred vision, and hot cheeks** (anticholinergic effect); he also complained of **palpitations** (due to arrhythmias).

PE

VS: tachycardia with irregular rhythm; **fever** (anticholinergic inability to sweat); hypotension. PE: patient **confused**; pupils dilated (MYDRIASIS); **skin warm and red; diminished peristalsis** with no peritoneal signs.

Labs

Lytes: normal. BUN and CPK normal. UA: **myoglobin** present. ECG: occasional premature ventricular contractions (PVCs) and **prolonged QRS and QT intervals**.

Imaging

CXR: no pathology found.

Treatment

Activated charcoal: hemodialysis and hemoperfusion are ineffective owing to large volume of distribution of TCAs: monitor and treat arrhythmias with $NaHCO_3$, lidocaine; treat hypotension with IV fluids or vasopressors if necessary.

Discussion

Tricyclic antidepressants (imipramine, amitriptyline, doxepin) block the reuptake of norepinephrine and serotonin and are used for endogenous depression treatment. TCAs are commonly taken by suicidal patients and are a major cause of poisoning and death. Intoxication or overdose may produce **seizures** and **myoclonic jerking** (most common clinical presentation) with **rhabdomyolysis. Death may occur within a few hours.** Other side effects are anticholinergic (**sedation, coma, xerostomia,** and **diminished bowel sounds**).

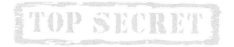

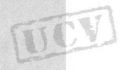
ID/CC   A 5-year-old male becomes **cyanotic** and has a **cardiorespiratory arrest** in the ER.

HPI   The child, a known asthmatic, had come to the hospital by ambulance 15 minutes earlier with severe **wheezing, intercostal retractions, nasal flaring, and marked dyspnea**. He was given inhaled corticosteroids.

PE   Immediate CPR was given, the patient was intubated, and assisted ventilation was administered. The patient came out of the arrest but then returned to his preadmission state of wheezing and respiratory failure.

Labs   CBC: **leukocytosis** (16,000) with neutrophilia. ABGs: mixed respiratory and metabolic acidosis with hypoxemia and hypercapnia. **Peak expiratory flow rate (PEFR) markedly reduced** (indicates severe airway obstruction).

Imaging   CXR: left lower lobe infiltrate compatible with pneumonia.

Treatment   Metaproterenol by inhalation until bronchospasms stop. Treat infection, acid-base/electrolyte imbalance.

Discussion   In a severe case of asthma such as this, a preexisting infection is usually the precipitating event. Inhaled steroids have no place in the treatment of an acute attack, as is also the case with sodium cromolyn (cromolyn prevents the release of mast cell mediators, useful for prophylaxis). IV steroids may be given but may take several hours to take full effect (they block leukotriene synthesis by blocking synthesis of phospholipase A2). **Inhaled beta-agonists are the mainstay of acute, emergent therapy** (they activate adenyl cyclase and thereby increase cAMP, which relaxes bronchial smooth muscle). Adverse effects include arrhythmias, tachycardia, and tremors.

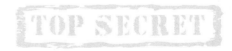

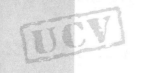

CASE 91

ID/CC

A 42-year-old female presents to her family doctor because of increasing concern over a **facial rash** for the last 2 months that cannot be concealed with cosmetics.

HPI

She has also noticed **joint pains** in the knees and sacral region as well as diarrhea. For the past 6 months, she has been treated with **procainamide** for a supraventricular arrhythmia.

PE

Hyperpigmented, brownish **butterfly rash** over the malar region. Left lung is hypoventilated, with dullness to percussion and decreased fremitus (PLEURAL EFFUSION); there is also a pericardial friction rub (due to pericarditis).

Labs

Increased **antinuclear antibody (ANA) titer**. Positive antihistone antibodies UA: **proteinuria** (> 0.5 mg/dL/day); presence of **cellular casts**. ECG: S-T, T-wave changes (suggestive of pericarditis).

Imaging

CXR: small left pleural effusion and enlargement of cardiac silhouette (due to pericardial effusion).

Treatment

Discontinue procainamide therapy and consider other class IA anti-arrhythmics. Lupus-like symptoms typically resolve.

Discussion

Approximately **one-third of patients** on **long-term procainamide** treatment develop a **lupus-like syndrome**. ANA titer is elevated in nearly all patients receiving this drug, which can also induce **pericarditis, pleuritis**, and pulmonary disease. Other adverse effects include rash, **fever, diarrhea, hepatitis**, and **agranulocytosis**. SLE-like syndrome can also be produced by penicillamine, **hydralazine** and **isoniazid**.

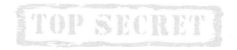

RHEUMATOLOGY

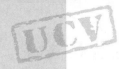

CASE 92

ID/CC A 30-year-old man is brought to the emergency room in a **stuporous** state with nausea, **protracted vomiting**, and malaise.

HPI He had been overtreating himself with Tylenol (acetaminophen) with up to 30 pills a day to relieve the pain and discomfort associated with a whiplash neck injury he sustained approximately a week ago.

PE VS: normal. PE: **icterus**; **asterixis**; patient **confused** and **dehydrated**; funduscopic exam normal.

Labs Markedly **elevated serum transaminases**; **elevated serum bilirubin**; **prolonged PT**; mildly elevated serum creatinine and BUN; mild hypoglycemia. ABGs: **metabolic acidosis. Serum acetaminophen levels in toxic range**.

Imaging CXR: within normal limits.

Micro Pathology Liver biopsy reveals overt coagulative centrilobular necrosis; cells appear shrunken and pyknotic with marked presence of neutrophils.

Treatment **N-acetylcysteine as a specific antidote** to replete hepatic glutathione levels; supportive management of fulminant hepatic and renal failure; consider liver transplant in severe cases.

Discussion One of the products of cytochrome P450 metabolism of acetaminophen is hepatotoxic. This reactive metabolite is normally detoxified by glutathione in the liver, but in large doses it may overwhelm the liver's capacity for detoxification. Renal damage may occur because of metabolism by the kidney. Encephalopathy, coma, and death may occur without treatment.

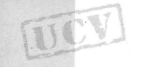

CASE 93

ID/CC
A 61-year-old male is admitted to the internal medicine ward for evaluation of **weight loss** and an **increase in abdominal girth**.

HPI
He is the father of an African student who is currently studying in the United States. His son brought him here from Central **Africa** for treatment of his disease.

PE
Thin, emaciated male; marked **jaundice**; abdomen markedly enlarged due to **ascitic fluid**; **hepatomegaly**; pitting **edema** in both lower legs.

Labs
CBC: anemia (Hb 6.3) (sometimes there may be polycythemia due to ectopic erythropoietin secretion). Increased α-fetoprotein; hypoglycemia (due to increased glycogen storage); AST and ALT elevated; alkaline phosphatase elevated.

Imaging
US/CT, abdomen: enlargement of liver with multiple nodularities involving the vena cava; enlargement of regional lymph nodes.

Micro Pathology
Liver biopsy confirms clinical diagnosis, showing fibrotic changes and glycogen accumulation with vacuolation and multinucleated giant cells; pleomorphic hepatocytes seen in a trabecular pattern (may also be adenoid or anaplastic) with malignant change (hepatocellular carcinoma).

Treatment
Palliative.

Discussion
Hepatocellular carcinoma is frequently seen in association with hepatitis B virus infections and with cirrhosis. There is a dramatic predisposition to this neoplasia in Africa and in parts of Asia; it is the most common visceral neoplasm in African men. Causative theories include the carcinogenic action of aflatoxins on genetically susceptible individuals and inactivation of the p53 tumor suppressor gene. Aflatoxins are produced by the contamination of peanuts and improperly stored grains (staple food in many African countries) with the fungus *Aspergillus flavus*.

TOXICOLOGY

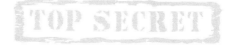

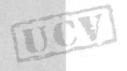

CASE 94

ID/CC   A 47-year-old obese male who has been a heavy smoker for 20 years (with COPD) visits his family doctor complaining of malaise, lack of appetite (ANOREXIA), and persistent **pain in his shoulders and lower back** together with **dyspnea and dizziness.**

HPI   He recently had a recurrence of gastroesophageal reflux disease, and nothing but his **aluminum gel** relieves it, so he has been taking large quantities of it in order to relieve his symptoms.

PE   Obese and **lethargic**; heart sounds with no murmurs; lungs have a few scattered rales in both bases; **petechial hemorrhages** in legs and arms.

Labs   CBC: mild **hemolytic anemia** (increased erythrocyte fragility); platelet count normal (but there are abnormalities in function-adhesion). **Phosphorus serum level low**; increased LDH.

Imaging   XR: no sign of osteomalacia (acute phosphorus deficiency, not chronic).

Treatment   Phosphorus supplements and/or switch to other antacids or H_2 receptor blockers; in severe cases, **deferoxamine** is used to chelate aluminum.

Discussion   Aluminum salts (HYDROXIDE) are used as antacids in many preparations. They commonly produce **constipation**, which is why most compounds add magnesium for its laxative properties to counteract the effects of aluminum. Another side effect of aluminum therapy is **impaired absorption of phosphorus in the GI tract**. With diminished available phosphate, the concentration of 2,3-diphosphoglycerate (2,3-DPG) decreases, leading to abnormal tissue oxygenation (malaise, dyspnea) and muscle weakness (including respiratory muscles). Hypophosphatemia, if persistent, may lead to osteomalacia.

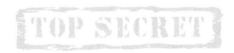

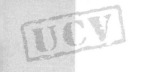

CASE 95

ID/CC

A 48-year-old factory worker is brought to the ER after a **chemical spill** because of **difficulty breathing** and **irritation of the eyes and throat**.

HPI

He denies allergies, previous surgical operations, diabetes, high blood pressure, infectious diseases, trauma, blood transfusions, and hospitalizations, and he is not on any current medication.

PE

VS: normal. PE: patient conscious, alert, oriented, and in no acute distress; **ammonia smell** emanating from clothes; **marked hyperemia** of ocular conjunctiva and upper respiratory passageways; throat mucosa and tongue **edematous** with mucosal **sloughing** on the left side; no laryngospasm; lungs clear to auscultation; abdomen is soft with no masses or peritoneal signs; no focal neurologic signs.

Labs

CBC/Lytes: normal. US: normal.

Imaging

CXR: no evidence of pneumomediastinum (seen with esophageal perforation with ammonia ingestion).

Treatment

Treatment depends on route of exposure to ammonia gas. Observe patient for upper airway obstruction due to inhalation injuries. For eyes and skin, wash exposed regions with water or saline. There are no specific antidotes for this or other caustic burns.

Discussion

Ammonia is used as a fertilizer, household chemical, and commercial cleaning agent. Ammonia gas is highly water soluble and produces its **corrosive effects** on contact with tissues such as the eyes and respiratory tract, producing severe laryngitis and tracheitis with possible laryngospasm.

TOXICOLOGY

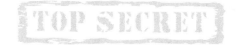

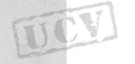
ID/CC A 10-year-old boy living near a pigment-manufacturing industry presen with a **burning sensation** in a **glove-and-stocking distribution** togeth with severe **bilateral arm and leg weakness**.

HPI He also presents with **hyperpigmentation** and thickening of the skin ove his palms and soles. The child is in the habit of **eating paint**.

PE Hyperkeratosis on palms and soles; peculiar "**raindrop**" **depigmentatio Aldrich-Mees lines** over nails; neurologic exam reveals decreased sens tion, decreased motor strength, absent deep tendon reflexes, and wasti (SYMMETRIC POLYNEUROPATHY) in arms and legs.

Labs **Arsenic levels** elevated **in blood, urine, and hair.**

Treatment **Chelation** with BAL; DMSA, or penicillamine.

Discussion Arsenic is used in a variety of settings, e.g., as pesticides, herbicides, ar rat poison and in the metallurgic industry. The intoxication may be acut with violent diarrhea, liver and renal necrosis, and shock potentially lea ing to death. In chronic exposure, the neurologic symptoms predomina over the gastrointestinal symptoms. The liver and kidney are also affecte in chronic exposure.

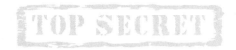

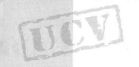

CASE 97

ID/CC

A 37-year-old male is brought to the ER by ambulance after collapsing while at work at a **metal-plating** factory.

HPI

The factory routinely uses **cyanide**-containing compounds in its chemical plating process. A coworker reports that shortly before the patient collapsed, he complained of feeling **nauseated** and having a **headache**.

PE

VS: tachycardia (HR 165); hypotension (BP 90/50). PE: patient is experiencing **agonal respiration**, is unresponsive to external stimuli, and exudes a bitter **almond odor**.

Labs

Measured venous oxygen saturation elevated (due to markedly decreased oxygen uptake).

Treatment

Treat all cyanide exposure as life-threatening. Give supplemental oxygen. Cyanide antidotes consist of amyl and sodium nitrates, which produce CN-scavenging compounds (especially methemoglobin). Sodium thiosulfate accelerates the conversion of cyanide to thiocyanate.

Discussion

Cyanide, one of the most powerful poisons known, is a chemical asphyxiant that binds to cytochrome oxidase, blocking the use of oxygen and producing fulminant tissue hypoxia and death in seconds if inhaled or in minutes if ingested. It is used in the photographic, shoe polish, fumigation, and metal-plating industries. Free cyanide is metabolized to thiocyanate, which is less toxic and easily excreted in the urine. Exposure to cyanide gas can be rapidly fatal; however, toxicity due to ingestion of cyanide salts can be slowed with delayed absorption in the GI tract. Administer activated charcoal if accidental oral ingestion is suspected.

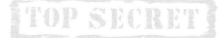

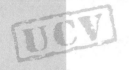

CASE 98

ID/CC   A 25-year-old male with **HIV/AIDS** complains of severe **shooting pain** in both lower extremities.

HPI   The patient is currently taking two **nucleoside reverse transcriptase inhibitors: didanosine (ddI)** and stavudine (d4T), as well as indinavir (a protease inhibitor).

PE   VS: normal. PE: **thin, cachectic** appearance; no evidence of sensory or motor deficits on neurologic exam.

Labs   CBC: leukopenia; elevated MCV (associated with taking reverse transcriptase inhibitors). LFTs mildly elevated.

Treatment   Discontinue ddI and/or d4T and replace with **non-nucleoside reverse transcriptase inhibitor** such as nevirapine. Analgesics, narcotics, tricyclic antidepressants, gabapentin, or alternative therapies such as acupuncture may be effective in treating peripheral neuropathy.

Discussion   Didanosine is a nucleoside reverse transcriptase inhibitor used in HAART (highly active antiretroviral therapy) for HIV/AIDS. Its main side effects are **dose-related peripheral neuropathy**, diarrhea, abdominal pain, and **pancreatitis** (1% to 10% risk). Didanosine is also associated with **increased liver enzymes** and **hyperuricemia**. It decreases absorption of numerous antibiotics, including ketoconazole, tetracycline, and fluoroquinolones, and concurrent administration is not recommended.

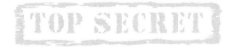

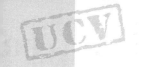
ID/CC

A 6-year-old boy is brought to the ER because of **slurred speech, lethargy** and **severe vomiting.** The patient was "helping" his father in the garage when he saw an **antifreeze** bottle and, out of curiosity, drank it.

HPI

On arrival at the local pediatric emergency room, the boy started having tonic-clonic **seizures.**

PE

VS: tachycardia (HR 108); no fever; **hypotension** (BP 80/40). PE: **hyper-ventilating** and experiencing **convulsions.**

Labs

CBC: leukocytosis (13,000). **Ethylene glycol found in blood; metabolic acidosis with elevated** osmolar and **anion gap.** Lytes: hyponatremia; hyperkalemia. BUN and creatinine levels normal. ECG: **premature ventricular beats.**

Imaging

CXR: no evidence of bronchoaspiration of ethylene glycol.

Treatment

Administer **ethanol** to saturate alcohol dehydrogenase, which prevents metabolism of ethylene glycol to its toxic metabolites. Administer **pyridoxine, folate, and thiamine** (to attenuate the effects of toxic metabolites). Treat convulsions with diazepam and monitor vital signs. **Hemodialysis** can effectively remove ethylene glycol and correct acidosis and electrolyte abnormalities.

Discussion

Ethylene glycol is the predominant component of antifreeze and may be used by alcoholics as an alcohol substitute. Because of its **sweet taste,** children and pets frequently ingest antifreeze. Its by-products may cause **metabolic acidosis, renal failure** (due to **intratubular deposition of oxalate crystals**), and death.

TOXICOLOGY

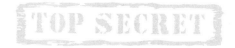

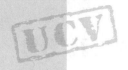

CASE 100

ID/CC   A 2-year-old male is brought to the emergency room by his mother after a bout of **vomiting**.

HPI   The child has been seen by ER staff physicians in the past for **numerous episodes of vomiting and diarrhea**.

PE   VS: **tachycardia** (HR 140); mild **hypotension** (BP 100/60). PE: **hyporeflexia; muscle weakness**, and tenderness.

Labs   Lytes: serum **potassium low**. BUN, CPK, and creatinine normal. ECG: no arrhythmias or conduction disturbances.

Treatment   Treat fluid and electrolyte imbalances. Monitor ECG for changes and possible **arrhythmias** (cause of death).

Discussion   Ipecac syrup is an effective drug when induction of vomit is necessary due to ingestion of drugs and poisons, mainly in children. The safety margin is wide, but deaths have occurred when **fluid extract** of ipecac has been administered (much more concentrated than ipecac syrup). Chronic ipecac poisoning should be suspected in cases in which children are repeatedly brought in with symptoms such as these. Reports of such misuse in cases of "Munchausen's syndrome by proxy" have been recorded. Intoxication may result in cardiomyopathy and fatal arrhythmia (ipecac contains emetine).

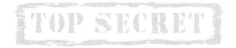

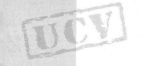

CASE 101

ID/CC
A 5-year-old male is brought to a medical clinic because of an episode of sudden, **vigorous vomiting** with no previous nausea (PROJECTILE VOMITING) (due to encephalopathy); his mother adds that the child has been **behaving strangely** and has been **irritable**.

HPI
He also complains of **weakness in his hands and feet**. The boy lives in an **old house** that was recently renovated (old residential **paints and house dust** may contain toxic amounts of lead). He has had episodes of abdominal pain in the past.

PE
Pallor; lethargy; **foot drop** (due to peripheral neuropathy); retinal stippling; lines in gums (LEAD LINES) (due to perivascular lead sulfide accumulation); **wasting of muscles of hand with motor weakness** (hand grip 50%).

Labs
CBC: hypochromic, microcytic anemia with basophilic stippling. Hyperuricemia. UA: **increased urinary coproporphyrin and aminolevulinic acid. Blood lead** and **free erythrocyte protoporphyrin levels elevated**; glycosuria; **hypophosphatemia**.

Imaging
XR, long bones: **broad bands** of **increased density** at metaphysis.

Gross Pathology
Marked edema of brain; peripheral nerve segmental demyelinization.

Micro Pathology
Acid-fast intranuclear inclusion bodies in renal tubular cells, hepatocytes, and osteoclasts; bone marrow biopsy shows **sideroblastic picture**.

Treatment
Separation from source of exposure; chelation therapy with CaEDTA or dimercaprol (IM), or by DMSA (succimer) or penicillamine (oral).

Discussion
Lead poisoning may be caused by gasoline, eating flaking wall paint (as occurs in pica), or using clay utensils with leaded glaze. Poisoning is more common in summer due to sun exposure with increased circulating porphyrins. Lead binds to disulfide groups, causing denaturation of enzymes, and inhibits ferrochelatase and δ-aminolevulinic acid dehydratase, thereby interfering with iron utilization in heme synthesis.

TOXICOLOGY

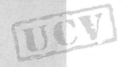

CASE 102

ID/CC
A 28-year-old male, a professor of chemistry at the local high school comes to the emergency room complaining of acute **retrosternal and epigastric pain** and frequent **vomiting** of blood-tinged material.

HPI
He admits to a **suicide attempt** through the ingestion of several teaspoons of **mercurium bichloride** (corrosive) from his chemistry lab. On arrival at the ER he had a **bloody, diarrheic** bowel movement.

PE
VS: **hypotension**; tachycardia. PE: pallor; skin cold and clammy; tongue whitish; patient is confused, **oliguric, and dyspneic**; moderate abdominal tenderness; **grayish discoloration of buccal mucosa**.

Labs
Elevated serum creatinine and BUN. UA: presence of tubular casts. Fractional excretion of sodium markedly increased; serum hemoglobin levels markedly elevated.

Gross Pathology
Acute tubular necrosis; acute irritative colitis with mucosal necrosis with sloughing and hemorrhage.

Treatment
Chelation therapy with dimercaprol, penicillamine, and succimer (DMSA); supportive management of acute tubular necrosis; GI decontamination for acute exposure to organic or inorganic mercury.

Discussion
Mercury, in its multiple forms, is toxic to human beings. Organic mercury is the most toxic. Acute toxicity is exemplified by this case. Chronic mercury exposure produces **proteinuria, stomatitis,** and **CNS signs,** mostly in children. These signs include insomnia, irritability, ataxia, nystagmus, and convulsions.

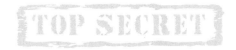

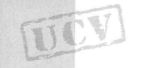

CASE 103

ID/CC	A 46-year-old **homeless alcoholic** is brought to the ER by two of his friends in a **confused, incoherent state**; he has been in the ER on many previous occasions.
HPI	He appears unkempt and, as usual, **smells heavily of alcohol**. He complains of nausea, vomiting, and abdominal pain, is very anxious, and constantly repeats that he **cannot see clearly**.
PE	VS: tachycardia; BP normal; **tachypnea** (respiratory compensation to severe acidosis). PE: patient confused as to time, person, and place; speech incoherent; no meningeal or peritoneal signs; no focal neurologic deficit; **marked photophobia** when eye reflex is elicited; papilledema.
Labs	CBC/Lytes: normal. Amylase normal (methanol may produce an acute pancreatitis). LFTs: slightly altered (due to chronic alcoholic liver disease). LP: CSF normal. ABGs: **pH 7.2** (ACIDOSIS). **Anion gap increased; serum osmolarity elevated** (due to osmotically active methanol). ECG: normal.
Imaging	CXR: normal. CT, brain: normal.
Micro Pathology	Retinal edema with degeneration of ganglion cells; optic nerve atrophy after acute event has subsided.
Treatment	Secure airway, breathing, and circulation; for severe acidosis, give sodium bicarbonate; antidote consists of an inhibitor of alcohol dehydrogenase such as **ethanol** or **fomepizole**; provide **folic acid** as a cofactor for formic acid metabolism; consider **hemodialysis** to remove toxin and correct acidosis.
Discussion	Methyl alcohol (METHANOL) is degraded by dehydrogenase to formaldehyde and formic acid, both of which are toxic compounds that cause a high-anion-gap metabolic acidosis together with ocular lesions that may lead to blindness (due to **retinal and optic nerve atrophy**).

TOXICOLOGY

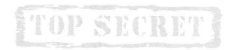

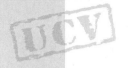

CASE 104

ID/CC

A 46-year-old girl scout guide presents to the emergency room of the local rural hospital with excessive **thirst**, weakness, protracted **vomiting**, **acute abdominal pain**, and **severe diarrhea**.

HPI

She has been in good health and states that during the camping trip she ate some **wild mushrooms** (about 6 hours ago) that she had hand-picked.

PE

VS: **tachycardia** (HR 165); **hypotension** (BP 85/40). PE: lethargy; disorientation; skin is cold and cyanotic; hyperactive bowel sounds on abdominal exam.

Labs

Liver transaminases and bilirubin elevated; PT increased; increased BUN and creatinine.

Treatment

Secure airway, breathing, and circulation; if patient presents within 1 hour after ingestion, consider gastric decontamination; thioctic acid may be useful as a free radical scavenger; **high-dose penicillin** blocks hepatic uptake of toxin and increases renal excretion; if hepatic failure ensues, orthotopic **liver transplantation** may be necessary.

Discussion

There are many species of toxic mushrooms, with clinical pictures varying according to the specific poison involved. Those most commonly involved in the United States are *Amanita phalloides* (delayed intoxication) and *A. muscaria* (rapid toxicity). According to mushroom type, toxins may produce anticholinergic effects (mydriasis, tachycardia, blurred vision) or muscarinic effects (salivation, myosis, bradycardia). These types of mushrooms are often picked and eaten by **amateur foragers**. Toxins are highly stable and remain after cooking. They are absorbed by intestinal cells, and subsequent cell death and sloughing occur within 8 to 12 hours of ingestion. Severe hepatic and renal necrosis is also a common effect of the toxins found in *Amanita phalloides*.

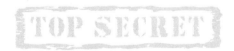

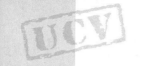

CASE 105

ID/CC A 33-year-old female with HIV/AIDS presents with a skin **rash**.

HPI Two weeks ago the patient was placed on triple antiretroviral therapy with AZT, didanosine, and **nevirapine**. She denies fevers, nausea, muscle/joint soreness, headaches, or abdominal pain.

PE VS: normal. PE: **nonpruritic, maculopapular, erythematous rash** diffusely spread across trunk, face, and extremities.

Labs CBC: leukopenia. LFTs mildly elevated.

Treatment Temporarily **discontinue or decrease nevirapine** dose and, if rash resolves, gradually **dose escalate** nevirapine to reduce risk of recurrence.

Discussion Nevirapine is a **non-nucleoside reverse transcriptase inhibitor (NNRTI)** that directly inhibits HIV reverse transcriptase and is used as part of a 3- or 4-drug regimen to treat HIV. Other NNRTIs include **delavirdine** and **efavirenz**. Side effects of the drug include **rash, fever, nausea, headache,** and **elevations in liver enzymes. Stevens-Johnson syndrome** is a rare but life-threatening complication. Since nevirapine induces **cytochrome P450**, it interacts with many drugs, including cimetidine, fluconazole, ketoconazole, azithromycin, and rifampin; taking such drugs with nevirapine may increase the risk of a rash.

TOXICOLOGY

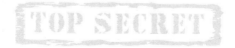

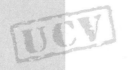

CASE 106

ID/CC   A 22-year-old white female who is a professional skier presents to the emergency room complaining of severe **malaise, dizziness**, jaundice, **very low urinary volumes**, and **fatigue**.

HPI   Following a recent skiing accident, in which she sprained her shoulder and knee, she took a total of 20 tablets of **diclofenac** over a 3-day period.

PE   VS: mild hypotension (BP 100/60); no fever. PE: severe dehydration; tenderness to palpation in epigastric area; **pitting ankle and palpebral edema**.

Labs   Lytes: **hyperkalemia**. Markedly **elevated BUN** and **serum creatinine**; urine osmolality increased; fractional excretion of sodium < 1%. UA: proteinuria.

Imaging   US, abdomen: normal-sized, normal-appearing kidneys.

Treatment   Volume replacement, metabolic correction, immediate withdrawal of NSAIDs, avoidance of all nephrotoxic medications.

Discussion   Use of NSAIDs, such as diclofenac can lead to acute renal failure via two mechanisms: (1) unopposed renal vasoconstriction by angiotensin II and norepinephrine; and (2) reduction in cardiac output caused by the associated rise in systemic vascular resistance (an effect that is opposite to the beneficial decrease in cardiac afterload induced by vasodilators). Thus, inhibition of prostaglandin synthesis by an NSAID can lead to **reversible renal ischemia, a decline in glomerular hydrostatic pressure** (the major driving force for glomerular filtration), and **acute renal failure**.

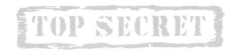

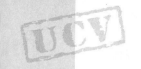

CASE 107

ID/CC
A 28-year-old male comes to his family medicine clinic and complains of **increased bruising** over the past 3 days, as well as **bleeding from the gums** while brushing his teeth.

HPI
The patient is an amateur weight lifter who recently tried to lift an excessive amount of weight but strained a muscle and has been **taking indomethacin** for pain.

PE
VS: normal. PE: athletic male with significant **ecchymoses** on chest and legs bilaterally; blood pressure cuff leaves petechial lines on arms; blood sample site taken on his arrival for routine blood work has become a large ecchymosis.

Labs
CBC/Lytes/UA: normal. LFTs: normal; **increased PT**.

Treatment
Discontinue indomethacin. Vitamin K may be used in patients with an elevated PT.

Discussion
NSAIDs inhibit cyclooxygenase 1 and 2 (COX-1 and COX-2), decreasing prostaglandin production and producing **analgesic**, **anti-inflammatory**, **antipyretic**, and **antiplatelet** effects. NSAIDs interfere with platelet function by inhibiting the synthesis of **thromboxane A_2 (TXA_2)**. Aspirin in particular is an irreversible inhibitor, and therefore the production of new platelets (about 8 days) is required before its anticlotting effects can be reversed. Moderate doses of NSAIDs can bring out subclinical platelet defects in otherwise healthy individuals.

TOXICOLOGY

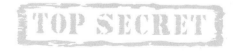

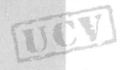

CASE 108

ID/CC   A 30-year-old **farmer** is brought to the emergency room with **sever** abdominal cramps and **vomiting**.

HPI   The patient is also **restless** and is **salivating profusely**. He has been working with a new pesticide for the past 3 months.

PE   Patient is nearly **stuporous**; **cyanosis** with marked respiratory distress **bilateral miotic pupils**; **marked salivation** and **lacrimation**; moderate dehydration; **hyperactive bowel sounds**; **fecal and urinary incontinence**

Labs   ABGs: marked **hypoxemia** with **hypercapnia**; uncompensated **respirator acidosis. Prerenal azotemia** on RFTs. Lytes: **hyperkalemia**.

Imaging CXR is normal.

Treatment Specific therapy includes administration of **atropine** (to offset cholinergic effects) and **pralidoxime** (chemically restores acetylcholinesterase administered early); supportive management for respiratory support an hemodialysis.

Discussion Organophosphates like parathion and carbamates are widely used a pesticides, and several nerve agents developed for chemical warfare ar rapid-acting and potent organophosphates. All of these toxins **inhibit th enzyme acetylcholinesterase**, preventing the breakdown of acetylcholine at cholinergic synapses. Whereas the **organophosphates may caus irreversible inhibition of** the enzyme, **carbamates have a transient an reversible effect**.

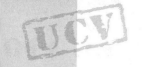

CASE 109

ID/CC

A 23-year-old female with **HIV/AIDS** presents to the infectious disease clinic for a regular follow-up.

HPI

She began antiretroviral therapy with AZT, ddI, and **nelfinavir** 1 year ago.

PE

VS: normal. PE: cachectic appearance with peripheral wasting and relative truncal sparing ("**lemon-on-stick**" appearance).

Labs

CBC: normal. Lipid panel reveals **hypercholesterolemia and hypertriglyceridemia; LFTs elevated.**

Treatment

Diet, exercise, and **lipid-lowering drugs** to reduce elevated cholesterol/triglyceride levels; monitor for onset of **diabetes**; consider **switching** or **discontinuing protease inhibitors** if necessary. **Human growth hormone** has shown limited benefit in the treatment of lipodystrophy.

Discussion

Nelfinavir, ritonavir, indinavir, and **saquinavir** comprise a class of anti-HIV drugs called protease inhibitors. Protease inhibitors are most potent when used as part of a 3- or 4-drug combination in patients who have never previously taken anti-HIV therapies. Side effects include **diarrhea, nausea, rash, lipodystrophy,** and **elevation in liver enzymes.** Lipodystrophy refers to changes in body fat composition that are believed to be related to protease inhibitor use. Other aspects of lipodystrophy include **elevated triglyceride/cholesterol** levels and **hyperglycemia** that can lead to **insulin resistance** and diabetes.

TOXICOLOGY

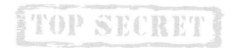

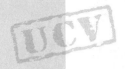
ID/CC   A 5-year-old female is brought by her parents to the pediatric ER with severe nausea, **hematemesis**, and **abdominal pain**.

HPI   She had been playing "candy maker" in her parents' room, and an **open aspirin bottle** was found on the floor. The child is otherwise healthy.

PE   VS: **marked increase in respiratory frequency** (HYPERVENTILATION); **fever**; BP normal. PE: flushed face; lethargy; **disorientation; dehydration**; **generalized petechiae**; abdominal pain.

Labs   CBC: **thrombocytopenia. Elevated PT**. Lytes: normal. ABGs: respiratory alkalosis and metabolic acidosis. Elevated blood salicylate levels.

Imaging   CXR: within normal limits for age.

Treatment If the patient presents early, consider **GI decontamination**; replace fluid losses and correct acid-base disorder; **alkalinize urine** to enhance excretion; if severe, hemodialysis may be necessary; treat gastritis with mucosal protectants, H_2 blockers, or proton pump inhibitors.

Discussion Aspirin toxicity may be pronounced in doses that are only five times the therapeutic amount. Decreased prostaglandin production results in decreased pain, inflammation, and fever. Acute ingestion may affect the integrity of the gastric mucosa and alter blood flow, which are prostaglandin-dependent processes. Diagnosis often depends on patient history, since quantitative levels are often not available. Salicylates stimulate the breathing center, thereby producing hyperventilation and respiratory alkalosis. Salicylates produce a metabolic acidosis as well as ketosis, so at different times during an intoxication and depending on the dosage, there will be different, often mixed, acid-base disorders.

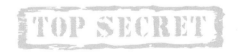

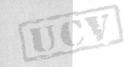

CASE 111

ID/CC

A newborn infant has **underdeveloped limbs** consisting of **short stumps without fingers or toes** (PHOCOMELIA).

HPI

Her mother took a drug for erythema nodosum leprosum, a severe complication of leprosy (HANSEN'S DISEASE) during the first trimester of an unexpected pregnancy; the drug was **thalidomide**.

PE

As described.

Discussion

Thalidomide is a well-known teratogen that was widely used during the first trimester of pregnancy as an agent for insomnia because of its quick sleep-inducing effect. It causes phocomelia, in which a child's limbs resemble the **flippers of a seal**, with failure of development of the long bones of the extremities. Several thousand children were born with this abnormality, making the medical community painfully aware of first-trimester teratogens. Thalidomide induces abortions and multiple other fetal abnormalities. Thalidomide, under highly regulated monitoring, is an effective treatment for complications of leprosy.

TOXICOLOGY

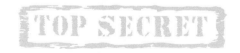

ANSWER KEY

1. Amiodarone Side Effects
2. Beta-Blocker Overdose
3. Captopril Side Effects
4. Digitalis Intoxication
5. Lidocaine Toxicity
6. Methyldopa Side Effects
7. Niacin Side Effects
8. Nitrate Exposure
9. Nitroglycerin Tolerance
10. Quinidine Side Effects
11. Verapamil Side Effects
12. Stevens–Johnson Syndrome
13. Vitamin A Toxicity
14. Anabolic Steroid Abuse
15. Cushing's Syndrome—Iatrogenic
16. Diethylstilbestrol (DES) Exposure
17. Insulin Overdose
18. Oral Contraceptive Side Effects
19. Osteoporosis Prophylaxis—Hormonal
20. Osteoporosis Prophylaxis—Nonhormonal
21. Osteoporotic Fracture—Bisphosphonates
22. Testosterone Deficiency
23. Alternative Pharmacotherapy
24. Anorectic/Anti-obesity Agents
25. Appetite Stimulants—Megestrol/THC
26. Cimetidine Side Effects
27. Hemorrhagic Gastritis—Drug-induced
28. Hepatitis—Halothane
29. Hepatitis—INH
30. Laxative Abuse
31. Pseudomembranous Colitis
32. Reye's Syndrome
33. Aniline Dye Carcinogenicity
34. Bleomycin Toxicity
35. Cisplatin Side Effects
36. Cyclophosphamide Side Effects
37. Doxorubicin Cardiotoxicity
38. Heparin Overdose
39. Iron Overdose
40. Methotrexate Toxicity
41. Warfarin Interactions
42. Warfarin Toxicity
43. Cyclosporine Side Effects
44. Interferon Use
45. Amphotericin B Toxicity
46. Chloramphenicol Side Effects
47. Chloroquine Toxicity
48. Drug Resistance
49. Fluoroquinolone Side Effects
50. Gentamicin Side Effects
51. Ketoconazole Side Effects
52. Penicillin Allergic Reaction
53. Rifampin Side Effects
54. Tamiflu Therapy
55. Tetracycline Rash
56. Zidovudine Toxicity
57. Loop Diuretic Side Effects
58. Renal Papillary Necrosis
59. Thiazide Side Effects
60. Tubulointerstitial Disease—Drug-induced
61. Viagra (Sildenafil) Therapy
62. Amantadine Toxicity
63. Anticonvulsant Osteomalacia
64. Carbamazepine Side Effects
65. Fetal Alcohol Syndrome
66. Ketamine Side Effects
67. Levodopa Side Effects
68. Malignant Hyperthermia
69. Parkinson's Disease—MPTP-induced
70. Phenytoin Overdose
71. COX-II Inhibitors
72. Amphetamine Abuse
73. Amphetamine Withdrawal
74. Barbiturate Intoxication
75. Caffeine Intoxication
76. Cannabis Intoxication
77. Clozapine Toxicity
78. Cocaine Abuse
79. Cocaine Withdrawal
80. Heroin Overdose
81. Lithium Side Effects
82. MAO-SSRI Interaction
83. MAO Inhibitor Hypertensive Crisis
84. Neuroleptic Malignant Syndrome
85. Nicotine Withdrawal
86. Opiate Withdrawal
87. Tardive Dyskinesia
88. Thioridazine Side Effects

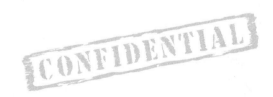

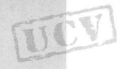

QUESTIONS

1. A news reporter traveled to an area where chloroquine-resistant *Plasmodium falcipartum* was prevalent. Before leaving on her trip, she took a drug for prophylaxis against malaria. Nevertheless, she developed an attack of malaria caused by *P. ovale*. Which drug do you suspect that she took for prophylaxis?

    A: Chloroquine
    B: Iodoquinol
    C: Mefloquine
    D: Pentamidine
    E: Primaquine
    F: Pyrimethamine

2. You're working in a busy clinic and an astute professor has been in for the third time with hypertension of 150–160/90–105. You correctly diagnose him with hypertension. He has no other diseases and asks you what is the evidence-based drug of choice for primary hypertension in him?

    A: ACE-I or beta-blocker
    B: ACE-I or diuretic
    C: Calcium channel blocker or ACE-I
    D: Calcium channel blocker or beta-blocker
    E: Diuretic or beta-blocker

3. Your patient presents to the office stating that he has been experiencing coughing and sneezing when he walks outside. After several examinations and laboratory analyses, you determine that he has allergies. Your patient is an airline pilot. In order to relieve his allergic symptoms you prescribe:

    A: Cimetidine
    B: Diphenhydramine
    C: Fexofenadine
    D: Metoclopramide
    E: Theophylline

4. Your patient is hearing voices and you want to start an anti-psychotic medication. Which of the following medications would require your very non-compliant patient to return to your clinic most frequently?

    A: Chlorpromazine
    B: Clozapine
    C: Fluphenazine
    D: Haldol
    E: Thiordazine

5. The half-life of a drug is longest in which situation?

    A: A small volume of distribution.
    B: A large volume of distribution.
    C: A high concentration of drug in the plasma.

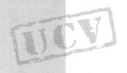

D: Low concentrations of the drug in organs and tissues.

E: If less total drug is present.

F: If an oral drug is given more frequently.

G: If an oral drug is given in higher doses.

6. You are seeing a new patient today in the clinic, they know they have a seizure disorder but do not know what kind of seizures. They are on phenytoin for prevention of recurrent seizure, which is the most likely type of seizure they suffer from?

    A: Absence

    B: Febrile seizure

    C: Grand mal seizure

    D: Myoclonic

    E: Petit mal seizure

7. A 52-year-old woman is referred to your GYN office with complaints of hot flashes and insomnia associated with menopause. She has a history of hepatitis B, hypertension, osteoporosis, chronic obstructive pulmonary disease, and hyperthyroidism. Of all her present conditions, which represents the only *absolute* contraindication to estrogen-based hormone replacement therapy?

    A: Chronic obstructive pulmonary disease

    B: Hepatitis B

    C: Hypertension

    D: Hyperthyroidism

    E: Osteoporosis

8. Current thinking is that the first line drug in treatment of congestive heart failure is which of the following?

    A: ACE inhibitors

    B: Beta-blockers

    C: Digitalis

    D: Diuretics

    E: Macrolides

9. A new patient presents to your office without complaints for a routine visit. This 50-year-old woman brought a list of medications to review with you. These medications include procainamide, propranolol, simvastatin, captopril, and sertraline. Which of the drugs this patient is taking can cause a lupus like syndrome?

    A: Captopril

    B: Procainamide

    C: Propranolol

    D: Sertraline

    E: Simvastatin

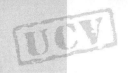
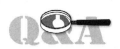

10. Your 64-year-old patient with congestive heart failure (CHF), hypertension (HTN), and diabetes mellitus type 2 (DM2) complains of seeing yellow-green haloes around lights. She is currently taking digoxin, hydrochlorothiazide, metformin, hydralazine, and glyburide. Which of these drugs causes the above side effects?

    A: Digoxin
    B: Glyburide
    C: Hydralazine
    D: Hydrochlorothiazide
    E: Metformin

11. You are called to the AIDS clinic one day to evaluate a young man who reports having difficulty with his vision for the past few days. Prior to entering the examination room you note that his last CD4 T-lymphocyte count was 37. After a careful exam your suspicions regarding his illness are confirmed. Which of the following is true about the drug choice used to treat this condition?

    A: It is one of the first drugs discovered to treat HIV.
    B: It is first triphosphorylated by viral tyrosine kinase.
    C: It is monophosphorylated by cellular enzymes.
    D: It is triphosphorylated by cellular enzymes.
    E: It inhibits host cell DNA polymerase.

12. A 40-year-old obese male with acanthosis nigricans and recurrent candidal infections of his axillary and groin regions has recently been diagnosed with type II diabetes mellitus. In treating this man, you want to take advantage of his endogenous insulin supply. Which of the following medication's mechanism of action is to stimulate the production of insulin in the pancreas?

    A: Pioglitazone
    B: Metformin
    C: Insulin
    D: Glyburide
    E: Acarbose

13. You are called to see a patient who has lost his pulse in the hospital. Rhythm strip shows a rapid rhythm which may be originating from the atrioventricular (AV) node. You recognize that a short-acting nodal blocker would be the best choice for this patient to possibly stop the arrhythmia. Which medication should be given?

    A: Propranolol
    B: Lidocaine
    C: Sotalol
    D: Epinephrine
    E: Adenosine

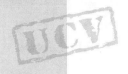

14. A 33-year-old female is brought to the hospital for acute mental status change by her husband. He reports that she has been taking the same medications for her anxiety and symptoms of paranoia for the past 5 years. On exam you find a diaphoretic woman who displays some rigidity of her extremities. Her blood pressure is 198/109. She also has a grossly elevated creatinine kinase. She is given bromocriptine, and she soon becomes more responsive. Which of the following medications could have caused this woman's very serious condition?

    A: Clozapene
    B: Dantrolene
    C: Fluoxetine
    D: Quetiapine
    E: Thiothixene

15. A 34-year-old female with a 12-year history of substance abuse from which she has now recovered is sent home by her dentist after having a cavity filled. Before going home she asks the doctor for a prescription for pain medications. If all pain medications had the same level of potency and would equally resolve her pain, which of the following pain medications would be the best option for her?

    A: Codeine
    B: Heroin
    C: Hydrocodone
    D: Morphine
    E: Tramadol

16. A 65-year-old African American male with a 3–4 day history of burning with urination and increased urgency presents to your clinic. His urinalysis is positive for white blood cells, leukocyte esterase, and nitrates. His CBC indicates that he is mildly anemic. He reports that his father and two brothers with anemia. In order to effectively treat his urinary tract infection while considering his family history which of the following antibiotics would be the best choice for this patient?

    A: Ciprofloxacin
    B: Erythromycin
    C: Nitrofurantoin
    D: Penicillin
    E: Trimethoprim-sulfamethoxazole

17. You are in the pediatric clinic doing a well-child check on an 8-year-old boy. He has a past medical history of asthma that is currently treated as needed (PRN) with albuterol, multidose inhaler. When asked, his mother tells you he has been using it daily for the last month due to increased shortness of breath. The most appropriate thing to do is:

    A: Add inhaled corticosteroids such as fluticasone on a daily basis reserving the albuterol for exacerbations only.

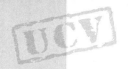
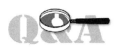

B: Add systemic steroids.

C: Congratulate them on using the albuterol as prescribed.

D: Stop the albuterol. He's outgrown his asthma.

E: Stop the albuterol. Prescribe only an inhaled corticosteroid.

18. A 15-year-old girl with a history of sexual and physical abuse has just lost four of her best friends in a motor vehicle accident caused by an alcohol-intoxicated truck driver. She has decided that life is not worth living and attempts to commit suicide by ingesting 25 individual 500-mg acetaminophen tablets at once. Without medical interventions, what is the method by which the patient is most likely to die? Choose the best answer:

A: Centrilobar hepatic necrosis

B: Centrilobular hepatic necrosis

C: Agranulocytosis

D: Drug fever

E: Pancreatitis

F: Skin rash secondary to an allergic reaction to the drug

19. Your first afternoon patient is a patient who you had diagnosed with depression but who was recently documented to be in a full manic phase. This appointment is to discuss the treatment options for the new diagnosis. You tell your patient that lithium is often used in treating patients with bipolar disorder, mania, and hypomania. Which of the following is true concerning lithium salts?

A: It is only effective in a small percentage of patients and is rarely used.

B: Its mode of action is clearly defined as a stabilization of the cellular membrane.

C: Lithium salts are very non-toxic and safe.

D: Lithium causes no noticeable effect on normal individuals.

E: Lithium is classified as a depressive.

20. You diagnosed Mr. S.L. with major depressive disorder 1 week ago and placed him on an appropriate dose of fluoxetine. He returns to see you today with the complaint "I've taken my medication but I don't feel any better Doc. My depression is just as bad as last week." What is the best treatment option for this patient at this time?

A: Increase the patient's dose of fluoxetine.

B: Reassure the patient that the medication takes several weeks to work and for him to be patient.

C: Reassure the patient that the medication takes several weeks to work and for him to be patient. Ask the patient if he is suicidal or homicidal at this time.

D: Start the patient on a second anti-psychotic.

E: Send the patient to the in-patient psychiatric ward for in-patient care since the patient is depressed and may harm himself.

ANSWERS

1. C

A: Chloroquine [Incorrect] One would not use chloroquine against chloroquine resistant species of *Plasmodia*.

B: Iodoquinol [Incorrect] This is a luminal amebicide. Iodoquinol may be used against *Entamoeba histolytica*, but not against any species of *Plasmodia*.

C: Mefloquine [Correct] Mefloquine is used for prophylaxis in cases where a patient is predicted to be exposed to chloroquine-resistant *P. falcipartum*, as in this case. This drug is a blood schizonticide, and has no effect on extraerythrocytic stages of the malarian parasite. Therefore, mefloquine does not act against *P. ovale* or *P. vivax*, which makes this patient liable to develop malaria through one of these species.

D: Pentamidine [Incorrect] This drug is used for trypanosomiasis and in *Pneumocystis carinii* pneumonia, but not against malaria.

E: Primaquine [Incorrect] Primaquine is used for prophylaxis in cases where a patient is predicted to be exposed to *P. ovale* or *P. vivax*. This patient was treated with a drug that would decrease her chances of getting malaria via *P. falciparum*. Primaquine is a tissue schizonticide and works by forming cellular oxidants.

F: Pyrimethamine [Incorrect] This is an antifolate drug that blocks folic acid synthesis in susceptible protozoa. This is a blood scizonticide that acts primarily against *P. falciparum*. This drug is not used for prophylactic purposes.

2. E

A: ACE-I or beta-blocker [Incorrect] While this is a very heated topic, currently diuretics and beta-blockers have shown greatest clinical efficacy in reducing MI, stroke, and CHF.

B: ACE-I or diuretic [Incorrect] While this is a very heated topic, currently diuretics and beta-blockers have shown greatest clinical efficacy in reducing MI, stroke, and CHF.

C: Calcium channel blocker or ACE-I [Incorrect] While this is a very heated topic, currently diuretics and beta-blockers have shown greatest clinical efficacy in reducing MI, stroke, and CHF.

D: Calcium channel blocker or beta-blocker [Incorrect] While this is a very heated topic, currently diuretics and beta-blockers have shown greatest clinical efficacy in reducing MI, stroke, and CHF.

E: Diuretic or beta-blocker [Correct] While this is a very heated topic, currently diuretics and beta-blockers have shown greatest clinical efficacy in reducing MI, stroke, and CHF.

3. C

A: Cimetidine [Incorrect] This is an H2 blocker, and would have no effect on allergic symptoms.

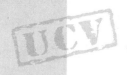

B: Diphenhydramine [Incorrect] This is an antihistamine that works by blocking H1 receptors. It would relieve the allergic symptoms that this patient is experiencing, but it has the greatest sedation effect of all the antihistamines. An airline pilot would not benefit from this type of relief as he would not be able to work.

C: Fexofenadine [Correct] Fexofenadine is an antihistamine that works by blocking H1 receptors. It possesses no sedation effects and thus would be appropriate for a patient like an airline pilot who needs to be able to stay awake.

D: Metoclopramide [Incorrect] Metoclopramide is a dopamine receptor blocker and a prokinetic agent. It has no effect of allergic symptoms that this patient is experiencing. Metoclopramide has antidopaminergic side effects like sedation, acute extrapyramidal symptoms, and elevated prolactin secretion.

E: Theophylline [Incorrect] Theophylline is a methylxanthine that works for nocturnal asthma treatment via slow release preparation by inhibition of adenosine receptor. It does not relieve allergic symptoms. Note: use this drug with caution as it has a very narrow therapeutic index.

4. B

A: Chlorpromazine [Incorrect] Clozapine is the only neuroleptic that clinicians must continually monitor for signs of bone marrow suppression and because of this it is not normally used as a first line.

B: Clozapine [Correct] Clozapine is the only neuroleptic that clinicians must continually monitor for signs of bone marrow suppression and because of this it is not normally used as a first line.

C: Fluphenazine [Incorrect] Clozapine is the only neuroleptic that clinicians must continually monitor for signs of bone marrow suppression and because of this is not normally used as a first line.

D: Haldol [Incorrect] Clozapine is the only neuroleptic that clinicians must continually monitor for signs of bone marrow suppression and because of this it is not normally used as a first line.

E: Thiordazine [Incorrect] Clozapine is the only neuroleptic that clinicians must continually monitor for signs of bone marrow suppression and because of this it is not normally used as a first line.

5. B

A: A small volume of distribution. [Incorrect] A small volume of distribution means that there is less total volume in the body that has the capacity to store the drug. Therefore, a small volume of distribution means more drug is going to be in the plasma and available for excretion or metabolism to a non-active compound.

B: A large volume of distribution. [Correct] A large volume of distribution simply means there is more available volume to contain the

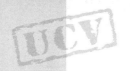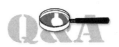

drug making it less likely to be eliminated by the kidneys or liver and extending the half life.

C: A high concentration of drug in the plasma. [Incorrect] The concentration of the drug has no effect on the half life.

D: Low concentrations of the drug in organs and tissues. [Incorrect] See above.

E: If less total drug is present. [Incorrect] This relates to the volume of distribution and the concentration in those tissues. It does not effect the half life.

F: If an oral drug is given more frequently. [Incorrect] You will not alter the half life if you give the drug more frequently or in higher doses.

G: If an oral drug is given in higher doses. [Incorrect] See above.

6.   C

A: Absence [Incorrect] Ethosuximide is the drug of choice for absence seizures.

B: Febrile seizure [Incorrect] This is often associated with high fever in children and treated with phenobarbital.

C: Grand mal seizure [Correct] Along with simple, complex and status epilepticus phenytoin is the drug of choice.

D: Myoclonic [Incorrect] Valproic acid or clonazepam are drugs of choice for Myoclonic seizures.

E: Petit mal seizure [Incorrect] This is also know as an absence seizure (see above).

7.   B

A: Chronic obstructive pulmonary disease. [Incorrect] Chronic obstructive pulmonary disease does not represent a contraindication to hormone replacement therapy.

B: Hepatitis B. [Correct] Liver disease along with pregnancy, breast cancer, endometrial cancer and a history of thrombophlebitis are *absolute* contraindications to estrogen based hormone replacement therapy.

C: Hypertension. [Incorrect] Hypertension is a potential side-effect of estrogen replacement but does not represent an absolute contraindication.

D: Hyperthyroidism. [Incorrect] Though estrogen replacement therapy increases levels of thyroxine-binding globulin, hyperthyroidism does not represent an absolute contraindication to therapy.

E: Osteoporosis. [Incorrect] Osteoporosis is actually helped by hormone replacement therapy because it reduces bone resorption.

8.   A

A: ACE inhibitors [Correct] ACE inhibitors have been shown to decrease vascular resistance, blood pressure, and increasing cardiac

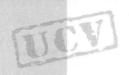

output. They also blunt the release of aldosterone and epinephrine caused by angiotensin two. Studies have shown ACE-I drugs to reduce the chances of arrhythmic death, MI, and stroke. Interestingly, studies are currently concluding to make new statements about ACE inhibitors and beta blockers so this may change in the future but currently ACE inhibition is the correct answer for this question and your patients.

B: Beta-blockers [Incorrect] Once thought to be counter-indicated in CHF, these medicines are now finding a place in the treatment of CHF and the prevention of further disease and complication. This is not first line.

C: Digitalis [Incorrect] Widely used in heart failure, it has no effect on mortality and is not used as a first line. It's utility is actually to decrease the number of hospitalizations of patients with CHF.

D: Diuretics [Incorrect] While useful in heart failure by reducing the effects of volume overload, decreasing the symptoms of paroxysmal nocturnal dyspnea and orthopnea it is not the first line.

E: Macrolides [Incorrect] This class of drugs, and all classes of anti biotics have not been shown to have any rewarding effects in the treatment of heart failure.

9.　B

A: Captopril [Incorrect] Captopril is an ace inhibitor. Its main side effects are cough, angioedema, and hyperkalemia.

B: Procainamide [Correct] Procainamide can cause a lupus-like effect Hydrazaline can also cause this side effect.

C: Propranolol [Incorrect] Propranolol is a non-selective beta-adrenergic antagonist. This class of drugs can cause depression, bradycardia bronchoconstriction, and sexual dysfunction.

D: Sertraline [Incorrect] Sertraline is a serotonin-specific reuptake inhibitor. SSRIs generally well tolerated with few adverse side effects.

E: Simvastatin [Incorrect] Simvastatin is an HMG-CoA reductase inhibitor, which is used in the treatment of hypercholesterolemia This class of drugs has been known to raise lever transaminase levels and cause myopathies.

10.　A

A: Digoxin [Correct] Digoxin is used for CHF and side effects include visual disturbances, nausea and vomiting, headache, fatigue and cardiac arrhythmias. Low potassium can potentiate toxicity.

B: Glyburide [Incorrect] Used for DM2 to stimulate release of insulin from the pancreas. May cause hypoglycemia, headache.

C: Hydralazine [Incorrect] Used for moderate to severe HTN and CHF Can cause a systemic lupus erythematosus (SLE) like syndrome

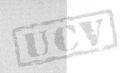
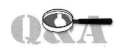

at chronically high doses. SVT can occur with intramuscular administration.

D: Hydrochlorothiazide [Incorrect] Used for hypertension. Side effects include hypokalemia, hyperglycemia, hyperuricemia, hyperlipidemia and hyponatremia.

E: Metformin [Incorrect] Used for DM2 to decrease hepatic glucose production and improve insulin sensitivity. May cause lactic acidosis, anorexia, nausea, vomiting, and rash.

11.   D

A: It is one of the first drugs discovered to treat HIV. [Incorrect] AZT (zidovudine) is one of the first drugs discovered to treat HIV.

B: It is first triphosphorylated by viral tyrosine kinase. [Incorrect] Ganciclovir is first monophosphorylated by viral tyrosine kinase, not triphosphorylated.

C: It is monophosphorylated by cellular enzymes. [Incorrect] Ganciclovir is triphosphorylated by cellular enzymes.

D: It is triphosphorylated by cellular enzymes. [Correct] This patient has CMV retinitis. The drug of choice to treat this condition is ganciclovir.

E: It inhibits host cell DNA polymerase. [Incorrect] Ganciclovir inhibits viral cell DNA polymerase, not host cell DNA polymerase.

12.   D

A: Pioglitazone [Incorrect] This drug does not cause further release of endogenous insulin. It is effective alone and in combination with other agents at increasing the body's sensitivity to insulin, particularly in the liver and skeletal muscles.

B: Metformin [Incorrect] This medication works primarily by decreasing the hyperglycemia associated with insulin resistance in the type II diabetic by reducing hepatic gluconeogenesis. It has been found to be effective alone and in combination with other agents in the treatment of type II diabetes. One of this drug's "side effects" is weight loss which is usually welcomed in the typical insulin resistant patient. It is also associated with severe lactic acidosis in some individuals.

C: Insulin [Incorrect] It is best to avoid putting a type II diabetic on insulin for as long as possible. In general, type I diabetics have a complete deficiency of insulin whereas type II diabetics may have too much insulin with an overall decrease in their insulin sensitivity. Increasing insulin in a type II diabetic who currently has elevated levels of insulin will not cause further secretion of insulin, nor will it resolve the problem of insulin resistance as the other oral hypoglycemic agents attempt to do. However women who develop gestational diabetes or who are type II diabetics prior to conceiving

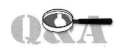

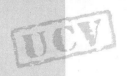

should be treated with insulin throughout the course of their pregnancy.

D: Glyburide [Correct] This is the classic oral hypoglycemic medication. It is a sulfonylurea and its primary action is to stimulate insulin release from the beta cells in the islets of Langerhans in the pancreas.

E: Acarbose [Incorrect] This drug works to decrease the intestinal absorption of starch and disaccharides. It has no effect on endogenous insulin release.

13. E

A: Propranolol [Incorrect] Although a beta-blocker with nodal blocking properties, propranolol is too long-acting and is not used in an emergency.

B: Lidocaine [Incorrect] Lidocaine is a sodium channel blocker without any significant effect on the AV node.

C: Sotalol [Incorrect] Sotalol is a beta-blocker that is also too long acting and not appropriate for an emergency. It may be used for atrial fibrillation.

D: Epinephrine [Incorrect] Epinephrine is an alpha- and beta-agonist which is likely to stimulate conduction through the AV node.

E: Adenosine [Correct] Adenosine is an extremely short-acting nodal blocker which is the treatment of choice for treating supraventricular tachycardias originating from the atrioventricular node.

14. E

A: Clozapene [Incorrect] This is an atypical antipsychotic medication. It has a decreased risk of causing NMS. The most worrisome side effect of clozapine is agranulocytosis. Patients on clozapine must have blood levels monitored at regular intervals.

B: Dantrolene [Incorrect] Dantrolene is a muscle relaxant that is useful in the treatment of NMS and malignant hyperthermia.

C: Fluoxetine [Incorrect] This is a selective serotonin reuptake inhibitor. It would be very unlikely to be the etiology of NMS in this patient.

D: Quetiapine [Incorrect] This is an atypical antipsychotic. It is a low potency medication and has less of a risk of causing NMS than the high potency antipsychotics.

E: Thiothixene [Correct] This patient is exhibiting the signs and symptoms of neuroleptic malignant syndrome (NMS). Thiothixine is a high potency antipsychotic medication; the drugs in this class have the established potential to cause NMS. This condition should initially be treated by discontinuing the offending agent. Subsequently, a dopamine receptor agonist, such as bromocriptine, should be added to decrease the extrapyramidal effects of the dopamine

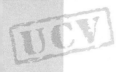
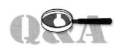

antagonist. It is also advisable to use a muscle relaxant such as dantrolene to augment therapy in patients with NMS.

15.   E

A: Codeine [Incorrect] This drug is a narcotic. Narcotics have an addictive potential.

B: Heroin [Incorrect] This drug is a narcotic. Narcotics have an addictive potential.

C: Hydrocodone [Incorrect] This drug is a narcotic. Narcotics have an addictive potential.

D: Morphine [Incorrect] This drug is a narcotic. Narcotics have an addictive potential.

E: Tramadol [Correct] This is the only *non*-narcotic drug on the list. A patient with a history of substance abuse (no matter what the substance of abuse was) must not be given medications that have the potential to be addicting and abused. The diagnosis of substance abuse is a lifetime diagnosis and patients once diagnosed, even if their addiction resolves, continue to maintain that diagnosis for life.

16.   A

A: Ciprofloxacin [Correct] The fluoroquinolones are very effective in treating uncomplicated urinary tract infections. This may not have been your first choice in an individual with a negative family history. However this patient is an African American man with several relatives with an unknown bleeding disorder, which is presumably G6PD deficiency. It would be advisable to avoid drugs which can precipitate this problem such as sulfa drugs.

B: Erythromycin [Incorrect] This is also a common therapy for treating urinary tract infections in the pregnant population, but would not be the drug of choice in this patient.

C: Nitrofurantoin [Incorrect] This is a bacteriostatic antibiotic frequently used to treat urinary tract infections in pregnant women, but this would not be the drug of choice for treating this older male's infection.

D: Penicillin [Incorrect] This antibiotic would not be effective against many of the gram negative bacteria which frequently cause urinary tract infections.

E: Trimethoprim-sulfamethoxazole [Incorrect] Although this would be a first line agent for most individuals, the risk of precipitating a G6PD crisis would warrant against using this drug in a patient with such a precarious family history. This medication is an effective 3-day treatment for uncomplicated urinary tract infections in men and in non-pregnant women.

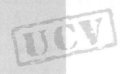

17. A

A: Add inhaled corticosteroids such as fluticasone on a daily ba~ reserving the albuterol for exacerbations only. [Correct] Using inhaled steroid as prophylactic medication is most appropriate this gives the best side effect profile.

B: Add systemic steroids. [Incorrect] The side effects of long-te~ steroid use are too severe to use steroids as a prophylactic medi~ tion. They may be used during an acute exacerbation for a sh~ period of time.

C: Congratulate them on using the albuterol as prescribed. [Incorre~ Albuterol is used only as needed, and should not be used on a da~ basis. Daily use indicates need for prophylactic medication.

D: Stop the albuterol. He's outgrown his asthma. [Incorrect] His asth~ has actually got worse, not better.

E: Stop the albuterol. Prescribe only an inhaled corticostero~ [Incorrect] Prophylactic use of inhaled corticosteroids is appropri~ However, most asthmatics need something for acute exacerbatio~

18. B

A: Centrilobar hepatic necrosis [Incorrect] The damage is in the c~ trilobular area.

B: Centrilobular hepatic necrosis [Correct] Toxic metabolites ~ acetaminophen are conjugated with glucuronic acid in the liver. ~ the presence of such a high concentration of acetaminophen, a~ therefore toxic metabolite, glutathione stores can be depleted. T~ leaves the toxic metabolite to bind to the hepatocellular constitue~ and results in hepatocellular damage. The most common area ~ damage is the centrilobular area of the liver.

C: Agranulocytosis [Incorrect] This is a possible serious reaction to ~ drug, but unlikely to kill her as the sole cause.

D: Drug fever [Incorrect] This is a possible but uncommon side eff~ of the drug if used at a therapeutic dose. But is not the most lik~ mechanism to kill her.

E: Pancreatitis [Incorrect] This is a possible serious reaction to ~ drug, but unlikely to kill her as the sole cause.

F: Skin rash secondary to an allergic reaction to the drug [Incorr~ This is a possible but uncommon side effect of the drug if used ~ therapeutic dose. But is not the most likely mechanism to kill h~

19. D

A: It is only effective in a small percentage of patients and is r~ used. [Incorrect] It is effective in 60–80% of patients with the a~ mentioned disorders; it is a highly utilized drug.

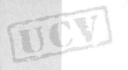

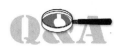

B: Its mode of action is clearly defined as a stabilization of the cellular membrane. [Incorrect] Lithium's mode of action is not known, it is theorized to be an alteration of the second messenger inositol triphosphate.

C: Lithium salts are very non-toxic and safe. [Incorrect] Lithium salts are very toxic and cause significant side effects in patients.

D: Lithium causes no noticeable effect on normal individuals. [Correct] Lithium is not known to cause any effect on normal individuals but still may cause many known side and adverse effects.

E: Lithium is classified as a depressive. [Incorrect] Lithium is not classified as a sedative, euphoriant, or a depressant. It is known as a salt or more simply an ion.

20.   C

A: Increase the patient's dose of fluoxetine. [Incorrect] This is not the best answer option. The patient will still have to wait several weeks until the effect of the drug is felt.

B: Reassure the patient that the medication takes several weeks to work and for him to be patient. [Incorrect] This is a correct answer but not the best option.

C: Reassure the patient that the medication takes several weeks to work and for him to be patient. Ask the patient if he is suicidal or homicidal at this time. [Correct] The SSRIs can take 4–8 weeks to show their effect. It is important to assess the possibility of the patient harming himself or others given that he may be frustrated with his medical condition and that he has not seen any results yet. If he is indeed suicidal that will warrant in-patient psychiatric care. If he is homicidal then further workup will be needed and may involve the duty to warn the person he has homicidal ideations toward.

D: Start the patient on a second anti-psychotic. [Incorrect] The patient is not on an anti-psychotic medication and displays no sign of psychosis to warrant placing him on one.

E: Send the patient to the in-patient psychiatric ward for in-patient care since the patient is depressed and may harm himself. [Incorrect] This patient does not need in-patient psychiatric care since there is no indication that the patient will harm himself or others.